Dr Ruth's Guide to

EROTIC AND SENSUOUS PLEASURES

Dr Ruth's Guide to

EROTIC AND SENSUOUS PLEASURES

DR RUTH K WESTHEIMER
& DR LOUIS LIEBERMAN

Robson Books

First published in Great Britain in 1992 by Robson Books Ltd, Bolsover House, 5–6 Clipstone Street, London W1P 7EB

Design by Sherrel Farnsworth

British Library Cataloguing-in-Publication Data
A catalogue record for this book is available from the British Library

Printed and bound in Great Britain by Hartnolls Ltd, Bodmin, Cornwall

To the brand-new addition to our family,
Ari Chaim Einleger,
a beautiful grandson whose smile is a joy
to behold—son to my daughter Miriam
and son-in-law Joel Einleger. Also
to my husband, Fred, and son, Joel,
with love and appreciation

R.K.W.

To my son, Joel David Lieberman,
who continually makes me proud of him,
and to Mary (Maria) Cuadrado,
the woman in my life

L.L.

My beloved is mine, and I am his,
that feedeth among lilies.

Until the day breathe, and
the shadows flee away,

Turn, my beloved, and be thou
like a gazelle or a young hart

Upon the mountains of spices.

The Song of Songs 2:16–17

And the man knew Eve his wife
and she conceived . . .

Genesis 4:1

Acknowledgments

Thanks are extended to the entire Shapolsky publishing crew—especially Isaac Mozeson and Sherrel Farnsworth—for a job well done in record time. Thanks are extended, as well, to our medical and other professional friends for their positive contributions and wisdom. Among our dedicated teachers, Helen Singer Kaplan, M.D., Ph.D., stands out above all others! Thanks, too, go to our trusting clients and creative students.

For advice and insightful suggestions, we thank Howard and Dr. Cynthia Fuchs Epstein. And to our many friends, only a few of whom can be listed here, go our thanks for your support, advice and contributions: Ron Alexander, Dr. Harold and Lois Alksne, Larry Angelo, Ruth and Howard Bachrach,

Susan Bakos, Mem and Zalman Bernstein, Dr. Mark Blechner, Susan Brown, Jerry Cohen, Dr. Finbarr Corr, Georgia Dullea, Betty Elam, Vincent Facchino, Jean and Dr. Robert Falzon, Dr. Jack Forest, Paula Fridgen, Harvey Gardner, Dr. Mike Glaser, Dr. David and Nancy Goslin, Fred Howard, Drs. Sam and Cynthia Janus, Alfred Kaplan, Bonnie Kaye, Philip and Bunny Kendall, Richard S. Kendall, Richard Korman, Dr. Nathan and Evelyn Kravetz, Rabbi and Mrs. Leonard Kravitz, Bill and Marga Kunreuther, Mitch Lebe, Joanne and Pierre Lehu, Rabbi and Mrs. Robert Lehman, John and Ginger Lollos, Diane Luckett, Sergeant Major Tom and Jo Luckett, Jeanette McDonald, Dale Ordes, Henry and Sydelle Ostberg, Fred and Ann Rosenberg, Cliff Rubin, Francine Ruskin, Rabbi Selig Salkowitz, Bernard Shir-Cliff, John A. Silberman, Dr. Raymond and Joy Simon, Elaine Silver, Fred Silverman, Dr. Arthur Snyder, Rudi Steinbach, Hannah Strauss, Eve and Oscar Stroh, Dr. William Sweeney, Greg Willenborg and Dr. Mildred Hope Witkin.

Ruth K. Westheimer and Louis Lieberman

Contents

CHAPTER 1

Sexual Pleasure Is Your Natural Right

"Another sex book? Who needs it? Aren't there enough on the market already?" We heard this from friends when we told them that we were planning a new book. These are fair questions, and friends always deserve an answer. So, to them and to you we say:

A. Yes, but this is a book about *better* sex,

B. You, you're the ones who need it, and

C. Yes, there are many other books on sex—but none deal with the subject as this one does.

This sex book does not focus exclusively on helping you overcome any sexual difficulties or problems. This book is for you even if you don't have any problems but merely want to improve the quality of your orgasmic response—or that of your partner.

Another unique aspect of this book is that we are trying to reach several different types of people. For example:

- There are those who, because of their upbringing, would have tremendous difficulties going to see a sex therapist and saying "I have a sex problem."
- There are men and women who have sexual functioning problems and do not want to talk about it at all with their partners, e.g., a woman who fakes orgasms. They would be afraid that their partner might find out if they went to a sex therapist.
- There are people who can not afford to go to a sex therapist or a clinic because they are often expensive.
- There are people who do not live near a clinic or a therapist.
- There are also those who want to avoid going to a sex therapist because they are hiding things from their sexual past or present—like having a lover.

We believe, therefore, that this book is different from both the sexual therapy guides and the sex manuals. Although its main thrust is "self help," we take the position that many apparent sexual dysfunctions may stem from the lack of learnable erotic skills. What appears to be a sex "problem" may, for some people, be reducible to the fact that there is just not enough erotic stimulation. This book was written to help you learn to become more erotically responsive and sensuous as part of the process of enjoying good sex and overcoming any sexual difficulties that you or your partner may have. We begin by helping you to enhance your erotic life before you even consider the possibility that *you* have a sex problem. You will most likely discover that you do not have as serious a sex problem as you think you have. Before we can work on any sexual dysfunctions, we will first help to ensure that you become more competent in the management of your erotic life and the conditions that permit the good sexual responses that you are capable of.

This brings us to a very important point of caution. If what we advocate does not work, we suggest that you see an appropriate and qualified doctor or therapist. Some problems require more or different kinds of attention and treatment than can come out of any book. You should always bear in mind that this guide is not the last place for you to get help. If a client tells a sex therapist, "You are the last resort" it is better for the therapy not to begin. There would be so much pressure on the client and therapist that no treatment method is likely to work. This is even more true if you are trying to get help from a book. One must always first believe that help is possible. We believe that hope and optimism are vital therapeutic aids in any doctor-patient relationship. So, take heart, there is help for you somewhere—for most of you right here in this guide to greater erotic and sensuous pleasures.

Why did we title this chapter "Sexual Pleasure Is Your

Natural Right"? Because many women, and some men too, do not *permit* themselves to have sexual pleasure. We find that they sometimes feel very uncomfortable about sex because they just don't feel that it's right. This problem may accompany any other problem that a man or a woman may have, and it may seem to be particularly prevalent in women. In Western Culture there has always been a lot of suspicion cast upon the woman who had strong sexual desires—even when she was married and the desire was only for her husband.

Up until a few decades ago, a woman with strong sexual desires that were not prompted by physical stimulation from her husband was likely to be considered a "nymphomaniac." This vague and now obsolete term was applied to all kinds of situations in which a woman's desires were of her own origin and where the need for orgasmic satisfaction caused her to be more assertive than women were supposed to be. Consequently, many women were made to feel guilty about something that was perfectly normal and natural. Even Freud, as much of a genius as he was, was subject to this widely held cultural view that the man was *supposed* to sexually stimulate the woman, to arouse her sexual excitement, but that she was not supposed to have these strong feelings on her own.

Part of the problem with Freud, of course, was that he was seeing patients who were already "sick," and generalizing on their behavior. (There is a danger even today when clinicians make broad generalizations based only on their patients.) In addition, Freud didn't have the physiological data on sexuality that we now have, based on the great work that Masters and Johnson did more than twenty years ago as well as on the significant contributions of Helen Singer Kaplan.

Some people like to take a cheap shot and blame religion for making women feel guilty about sex, but the anti-sexuality is more often to be blamed on society at large rather than on religious teachings alone. We know that many women have been brought up with the messages that only "bad" girls, "dirty" girls, "sinful" girls are involved in sexual urges and acts before marriage. But what happened to the perfectly normal, "nice" young women who did have erotic thoughts? They often began to feel guilty about these thoughts; so much so that strong messages of sexual repression were carried over even to their later married life. As we said in our last book, *Sex and Morality: Who Is Teaching Our Sex Standards?*, it is not that the message of Western religions is basically anti-sex, but that the way it is often presented to young people became distorted during the Victorian period so that many people began to sanctify their anti-sexuality under the long robes of religion.

But, luckily for us in the 1990s, we have the kinds of social, scientific, and historical information to put this anti-sexuality in perspective. When we note the "Scarlet Letter" disdain for sexuality during the Puritan period in this country, for example, we can now understand the increased necessity to preserve the family unit and to maintain self-discipline when faced with early America's sometimes chaotic environment. So, speaking in the name of their religion from the Old Country, people had to rail against all of those aspects of sexual freedom that might result in children born out of wedlock, venereal disease, adultery, and so forth.

What developed out of this societal control mechanism was an emphasis on sexual shame—because if a woman did get sexually aroused before or outside of marriage, there was nothing she could do for herself. A woman might then say to herself, "There must be something drastically wrong with me because I walk down the street and I think about sex." But let us look beyond our American attitudes. If we look at ancient Western societies (like the Greeks), and look at Eastern societies (like the Chinese, Japanese, or Indians) we find widespread acceptance of women's natural eroticism.

We also know that many men and women develop their shameful guilt feelings about sex from their early childhood when parents punished them for masturbating. This, too, we discussed in the *Sex and Morality* book, where we point out that sometimes such punishment results in poor self-image and poor body image development during adolescence. Too often this extends into later life and contributes to sexual dysfunction problems. We believe that it is very important for people to feel comfortable about touching their own bodies in order not to be "uptight" about locating their most sensitive erogenous areas and communicating their sexual desires to their partners.

Speaking of partners, they add another dimension of meaning to our chapter "Sexual Pleasure is Your Natural Right." Because sexual activity, except for masturbation, is an interpersonal act, your partner's right is your obligation. You are obligated psychologically as well as physically to be in the best state possible to both give and receive maximum pleasure. Of course, we are only speaking about persons who *choose* to have sex and who place a high value on sexual pleasure. Some persons may choose a lifestyle that includes celibacy, or even a marriage with little or no sex. That may be perfectly acceptable and healthy for them, but our book is addressed to the majority of people for whom sex is an important component of their interpersonal relations and emotional life. So once you have made that choice—and we hope that you will only have sex after reasoned choice rather than arbitrary passion, a drugged stupor, or being pressured into it—you then have the obligation to make that sexual relationship a happy and fulfilling one. Family stability and a commitment to raising healthy and happy children is the obligation of all of us who are parents. All too often, without realizing it, unexpressed sexual dissatisfaction causes couples to bring their anger from the bedroom to the rest of the house, just as we know that some people bring anger from elsewhere to their bed, resulting in bad sex. In either case, we will try to help you to keep stress and anger out of a loving sexual relationship.

We know that it may make some people feel nervous, self-conscious, or even silly when they consider doing the kinds of different exercises we will suggest in this book—especially if they were brought up to have strong negative feelings about sex, the body, touching oneself, and openly talking about sexual details. All we can say is: "Give this a try." We know that many men and women can't just plunge into different sexual behavior as a means of developing a better sexual experience. We therefore suggest a series of steps, starting with those with which you will feel most comfortable. We will then move on to things you can do by yourself that will help you appreciate your body in a non-sexual way. From there we will suggest ways to more directly use sexual aids that may enhance your erotic interest and behavior. Lastly, we will discuss how you can tackle the sexual problem you *think* you might have.

Let us conclude this first chapter with a brief description

of how this book is organized. In Chapters 2 and 3, we will define and describe the most common types of sexual dysfunctions and problems that people have. We will then have a common set of terms to avoid any more confusion than already exists among most people who discuss sexual problems. We will talk about those problems that are specific to men, those that are specific to women, and those that are common to both sexes.

Now, even though you may say: "Aha, so that is what my problem is," or "Hmm, I always suspected that he has this (or that) problem," *please, please,* try not to jump to such conclusions. We stress this caution, because, in our experience, we've seen many people link the wrong problem to the right symptoms. In reality, something else, something very easily handled, is often guilty of producing the same effect. In order to guide you to a more well-considered conclusion, we will discuss other things in Chapters 4 through 7—many of them involving changing of attitudes and settings as well as learning some erotic skills—which should be ruled out before arriving at the conclusion that you have a particular sexual problem. In Chapters 8 and 9 we will teach you how you can help yourself or work with your spouse (or lover) to help each other.

Can we guarantee that all your problems will be solved by this one book? Of course not! Some of you may have to go for additional work with a therapist, and we hope you will have gained sufficient insight by the end of this book to know if you do need a therapist. Even in that case, this book will have given you some additional erotic skills to work with, and a base of experience and knowledge to bring to your therapy.

This book will enable most of you to overcome the simpler kinds of sexual problems and certainly to enhance your sexual pleasure, regardless of your present situation.

CHAPTER 2

Women: What Are Your *Problems?*

How do you know that you have a sexual problem? If you want to have sex but cannot find a sex partner, that may or may not relate to a sexual problem. If you experience some discomfort or pain when you have sex, that may be more of a medical than a purely sexual problem. Even if you have lost most or all of your sexual desire, it may not necessarily indicate a sexual problem. What we are getting at with such evasive answers is that sexual problems are not always clear-cut or easy to define. But the good news is that the elimination of what you *think* may be a sexual problem may be easier than defining the problem. Read on to discover how something may and may not be a problem at the same time!

What we are focussing on in this book is the broadest possible definition of what a sexual problem may be: *if you are dissatisfied with any aspect of your sexual performance or sensation at any stage of the sex act (assuming you really care for your partner).* If we cannot suggest a way for you to solve your problem with the aid of this book, then we believe that you should seek the professional services of a qualified and accredited sex therapist for further analysis of the problem. But, give us a try first! You may be surprised with what you can do for yourself. Let us first look at the most common sexual problems of women who come to us for help. These are called "sexual dysfunctions," a technical term meaning that something is interfering with one's desired sexual performance or feelings. The most common of these sexual dysfunctions are:

- Orgasm difficulties
- Painful intercourse
- Lack of sexual interest

Other problems such as boredom with a sexual routine, the presence of children or in-laws who can hear through the walls, worries about the content of sexual fantasies, and so forth, are not sexual dysfunction problems at all. These require a little more sexual literacy rather than sexual treatment. Many of these kinds of problems have been dealt with in our previous books and we shall discuss some aspects of them in subsequent chapters here.

There are other kinds of sex problems that are deeper and that require the services of a psychotherapist before any real sexual behavior changes may take place. For example, we see many women who don't permit themselves to have any pleasure—sexual or otherwise. In one case an only child of a mother who lives far away came to see us because she had almost no sexual desires. She felt that to permit herself to have pleasure would be betraying her mother who does not have pleasure, who is alone and unhappy. Pleasure made her feel guilty. She fancied her mother thinking: "If I am not with you, how can you enjoy yourself?" For this kind of problem, she needed far more than the kinds of exercises and common sense presented in this book. She had to consult a professional therapist to be helped.

For some other problems, one may have to go to a physician. If you feel pain or much discomfort during intercourse, this may indicate a serious medical problem. The problem could be in your head or in your vagina, or in the way that you and your partner are having sex. In all cases the problem is real and must be dealt with if you are to enjoy the sex life you deserve. It must be quickly diagnosed and just as quickly treated.

Now, let us return to the three types of problems we listed above:

Orgasm Difficulties

Perhaps the most common concern regarding women's sexual performance is related to their orgasms. Do women *need* orgasms? This simple question needs a two-part answer. First, we know that once a woman is sexually aroused, the flow of blood to the labia, clitoris, and other parts of the genitals creates a tension that is best relieved through orgasm. Frequent sexual excitement without orgasmic relief has resulted, for some women, in various aches and pains as well as nervous tensions. And, besides, orgasms feel fantastic.

Now, for the second part of our answer: "So," some opponent of women's sexual pleasure might say, "if women never get sexually excited, they don't need an orgasm, right?" Wrong! While it is true that women may still conceive without experiencing orgasm, and they may feel a good deal of sexual pleasure, excitement, and satisfaction without an orgasm, they are clearly missing out on nature's bonus in the body. We support the view of those scientists who point out that the process of evolution (or God) has created a magnificent human male and female body, whose every part, system, and response has a reason to exist. To the female, as well as the male, was given the ability to have this marvelous sensual experience we call an orgasm. We can't help but believe that such a complicated reflex as this is there for a profound and beneficial purpose.

Some people, professionals and lay alike, have unfairly labelled women's non-orgasmic situation as an affliction. That is, if a woman had not yet learned to create the conditions or to receive sufficient stimulation to allow the orgasm reflex to occur, she might be called "frigid." And some husbands and partners have put an unfair amount of pressure on women, even out of loving consideration, to make sure they have an orgasm every time. So, please, you men out there: wait until you reach Chapter 9, where you will learn how to work *along with your partner* to reach the kind of orgasm *she* wants. Don't always be so egotistical to think that it is only the male who can bring the woman to orgasm. She has a part to play in all this too, you know.

Some letters we get are from women who are very certain that they are not having orgasms, while others are unclear. In most cases, women know very well if they are not having orgasms. Most women who come to a sex therapist with this problem say: "I am not having orgasms. Can you help me?" How do they know they are not having orgasms? In some cases, they had them some time earlier, but not now. In one case, a woman only had orgasms some years ago with a former lover. She knows by way of comparison.

Then again, take the example of another woman's problem. She feels sexual desire and she does get aroused— meaning lubrication, blood flow to the genital area, engorgement of the outer and inner labia, and an erection of the clitoris. She feels an excitement and she feels an urge to come to a resolution. She anticipates a lightning-and-thunder conclusion to all the feelings and sensations storming through her body—but nothing happens. Did she have an orgasm? She knows that she experienced more than the quickly passing sexual excitement of seeing a sexy guy walking by. When experiencing heightened sexual arousal the woman knows that if she does not have an orgasm she will feel uncomfortable and frustrated. She knows this by past frustrations. You see, the orgasmic resolution is something a woman feels must take place when there is *sufficient physical stimulation* to bring her to that point. Even a woman who has never experienced orgasm will feel this desire for resolution of this more intense sexual activity.

And it is not merely thoughts that bring her to this point. When a woman has a partner who gives her sufficient physical stimulation, or if she gives herself sufficient stimulation, then she will be quite aware of the sensation of not reaching orgasm. (In Chapter 8 we shall detail more fully what "sufficient stimulation" is.) A woman who consistently does not have any orgasms may be considered to be, at *present*, non-orgasmic. Being non-orgasmic is not a permanent condition and certainly not a sickness. It merely means that the right conditions or stimulations have not been met to reach the optimal sexual response we call orgasm.

When a woman is with a partner whom she basically likes, in an environment she enjoys (not in the back seat of a car where she worries), and with no legal, religious, or other outside restraints telling her she shouldn't "let go"—if all the conditions are right and she still cannot reach that peak, then we have a classic case of a non-orgasmic woman.

The illustrations above suggest that the "problem" of not having orgasms may be broadly classified into two types. One is where the problem is due to the inability of the partner to bring a woman to orgasm, and the other where no matter how sexually skilled the partner is, the woman just cannot reach orgasm. In order to treat the problem, as we shall show later, it is necessary to understand the conditions under which orgasms may or may not occur. A woman may be orgasmic with self-stimulation, but not with her partner. She may be orgasmic with one partner but not another. Or, neither she herself nor her partner can bring her to orgasm. Since these situations require somewhat different corrective approaches, a woman has to know which situation applies to her.

There is another type of orgasmic problem that we sometimes see. There are some women who do not know that there may be a "flat moment" preceding the orgasmic response when it looks as if nothing is going to happen. Many women say that they don't experience this at all. But other women, when they have this "flat moment" might think: "Nothing is going to happen, so I might as well forget about it." They then turn themselves off and their lack of faith becomes a self-fulfilling prophecy: "See, I can't have an orgasm." Now, whether this "flat moment" is a natural physiological stress reduction built in to the orgasmic reflex, or whether it is peculiar to some women is unknown, but a woman who experiences this "flat moment" should keep up the stimulation to get past this point.

If the woman is able to reach orgasm through self-stimulation, and/or if the woman had reached orgasm with a previous partner, it does not mean that she is subconsciously rejecting her present lover. It may indicate an inability to communicate to the man what kinds of physical pressures and movements she needs to reach an orgasm. And, the problem does not necessarily point to any sexual diffidence on the part of the man. But he can't guess what's on her mind. Remember the "World's Greatest Lover" may be so only in his own mind. He means well, but you must help him and educate him about the particulars of *your* body.

In order to get a clearer understanding of what is producing the problem, one of the things a woman must consider is the relationship she has with her husband or partner. All the sex therapy and advice in the world won't help those women who basically don't like the person they are having sex with. You must try to understand your true feelings about your partner, and make sure that you do indeed want to have sex with him in a loving and fulfilling way. If you don't, then you should see a marriage counselor, pastoral counselor, or some other professional who could help you resolve your interpersonal problems. Again, you must take control over the abiding conditions before you can have the kind of orgasm you want!

One special kind of orgasm difficulty we treat is really caused by the mass media and folk myths. We are referring to the idea that only young women are sexually attractive, and that when a woman gets older she replaces her interest in sex with sitting in the rocking chair and knitting for her grandchildren. Nonsense! It is merely a cultural stereotype that an older woman (or man) loses interest in sex. Not even the removal of the uterus or menopause results in significant decreases in sexual desire. You have to *will* yourself to lose interest by believing the myths. "Hot flashes," which often accompany menopause, are sometimes used as an excuse by women who don't want to have sex with their husbands for other reasons. We hear them say: "See, my body is now telling me that my sexual life is over." We tell them that these hot flashes do signal hormonal changes during menopause, but it definitely does not mean the end of your sexuality.

On the contrary, for many women now free of the concern for pregnancy and with the children out of the house, this is a time to celebrate the recovered privacy and intimacy that may have been buried for decades. Husband and wife can now have a ball like two newlyweds, if they so desire. Sexiness is all in your head and often a change in attitude is called for before there can be the desired change in orgasmic response. For some women, sex can be better than ever when they get older. Although the orgasmic response may be a little weaker, it can still be fantastic for you women into your eighties and nineties. And who knows beyond that? If you do know, please tell us about it.

Painful Intercourse

When we use the term "painful intercourse" we are referring to pain from two separate causes. One cause of pain in the vaginal area is the result of attempts at penetration. This pain may derive not only from the penetration of a penis, but also from a finger or even a tampon. The other cause of pain taken up here occurs *after* penetration of the penis.

What do we mean by pain and how much discomfort should a woman accept during the act of intercourse? The only safe answer we can give to these questions is that *any discomfort* a woman feels during intercourse has to be dealt with. Slight pain doesn't mean that the woman has a problem —it may be as simple as the position of the penis entering the vagina. On the other hand, any discomfort or pain, even when innocuous, will detract from the pleasure of the sexual act and may have harmful psychological consequences. Even a subconscious aversion to sex because of a *small* pain can lead to a broken relationship, something harder to mend than most medical or physical problems.

Of course, if there is a physical basis for the pain or discomfort, this must be attended to by a gynecologist as soon as possible. Use your good common sense. If the suggestions here don't alleviate the discomfort at once, consider the painful sex a symptom, not a cause, and see your gynecologist. Such difficulties must not be downplayed as just one more of the aches and pains of life. Even when a young woman is having intercourse for the first few times, there might be some slight discomfort or painful pressure upon penetration. If there is more than just a slight discomfort or if a slight discomfort lasts more than a reasonable number of coital acts, she must see a gynecologist.

Probably the most commonly felt pain upon and immediately following penetration occurs when the woman has not been sufficiently aroused to generate good lubrication in the vagina. In some cases the woman might naturally produce insufficient lubrication. If the pain seems only to be due to this, use a sexual lubricant such as K-Y jelly. Petroleum Vaseline should not be used if you are using a condom or diaphragm because it may cause deterioration of the contraceptive material. If the use of a lubricant does not prevent painful penetration, then a visit to the gynecologist is in order.

What about the situations where the man cannot penetrate with his penis? He may be able to get a finger in, but not the penis. It might be that his penis is unusually wide, and the couple would have to try a different position. (See Chapter 9.) Research has shown that the vagina is very elastic and can usually accommodate all penis sizes. Sometimes the problem lies in the woman's *perception* that the penis is too large. If she grew up conditioned to think of the penis as huge, "dangerous," or "disgusting," perhaps because of a childhood experience, she might involuntarily contract the vaginal muscle before penetration as a way of keeping it out. The resulting pain would have nothing to do with lack of lubrication or insufficient love for the man, but rather with a deeply rooted fear of the penis which must be treated by a clinical psychologist or psychiatrist.

Lack of Sexual Desire

We recently analyzed the letters that came to the different "Dr. Ruth" radio and TV shows as well as the "Dr. Ruth" newspaper columns. One of the interesting findings to come out of this was that a lack of sexual desire is one of the most frequent complaints of people reporting a sexual dysfunction. We found that almost a quarter (twenty-four percent) of all the people who said that they had a sexual dysfunction problem mentioned a lack of sexual desire—and this was equally divided between men and women.

In the past, medical people apparently didn't take much notice of this as a problem because it was just assumed that all men have this "naturally" strong libido, or urge to have sex, while women have to be aroused during loving foreplay.

Modern studies have found, however, that sexual desire is the natural outcome of one's *interest* in sex. Sexual desire, just like interest, may precede any kind of physical or psychological stimulation. In the vernacular, people use the term "horny" to mean a state of strong and sustained sexual desire. "Horniness" is that inner sexual feeling that doesn't need erotic stimulation and is the basic sensation upon which further sexual stimulation then builds. Sexual desire, then, is not something that someone gives you; it is worked upon and acted upon through sensuous and other kinds of stimulation and erotic behavior you may engage in even when you are by yourself. "Horniness" is the feeling women have that makes them want to have sex with their husbands as soon as they get home, or that urges them to go call someone listed in their address book for an intimate dinner and what follows.

The sex manuals of yesteryear were certainly well intentioned and romantic in orientation, but not very knowledgeable about the workings of sexual desire. The great work of Masters and Johnson, and then of Helen Singer Kaplan, revolutionized our thinking about sex based on their scientific research. We now know that all too many men and women deprive themselves of the pleasures of a loving sexual relationship, even within marriage, because they are "just not interested" in sex. That is, they prefer not to do anything about sex, even to think about it. In a sense, lack of interest in sex is the most extreme form of lack of sexual desire. Luckily, most people with this problem, who write to us, have *some* interest in sex, but no real passions, urges, or strong positive feelings about it.

What don't we mean by "lack of sexual desire"? Some people think this describes a woman (or a man), who experiences no orgasm or even sexual excitement after stimulation from a sexual partner or through masturbation. But that is not what we mean by it, because lack of desire is before the arousal stage, before the sexual interaction. It basically is, in its most extreme form, no desire to do anything at all about having sex. Let us give you a personal example from Dr. Ruth's life. My husband, Fred, and my friends are always trying to get me to use a computer. But I have no interest in computers; I am bored if anyone talks about computers around me. I turn away when someone shows me his/her new computer. I say, "That's nice," with no interest or sincerity in my voice. If I never saw another computer in my life I would be just as happy. This doesn't mean that I couldn't operate a computer if I had to, but that I prefer to avoid them. In other words, not only do I have no desire to operate a computer, I have no interest in the subject at all! Extreme, you say, but that is exactly how some people feel about sex. They couldn't care less!

Do not confuse lack of orgasmic response with lack of sexual desire. The lack of desire is, in varying degrees, the lack of interest—a problem of the mind, not the genitals. When you have no interest at all, you don't even put yourself in the position where you have to behave sexually. When you have some interest, but very little desire, you may act very passively and wait until your partner takes the initiative. Some people have suggested that the lack of desire is the result of the way some women have been brought up in our Western Culture. That is, they are taught to suppress their sexual feelings until "aroused" by a man. The paradox is that some women who complain of lack of sexual desire may be easily able to reach orgasm, while other women who have a great deal of sexual interest and desire may still be non-orgasmic. Where is it written that sex is simple to understand?!

We have seen a number of cases where women, married for many years in some cases, married because it was the right time and because the men seemed like potentially good husbands and fathers. Or, they might have been marriages of convenience or "arranged" marriages. These women knew that they were expected to have intercourse, and even though they had no desire for sex, they knew that it would create conflict if they didn't carry out their part of the marital contract. So they went through the motions without ever enjoying it. This does not mean that they did not care for or love their husbands, but that the element of passion was missing. Many of these women realized that something was wrong, but they did not want to risk their marriages by confronting their feelings.

Their sexual performance may have been perfectly adequate. They lubricated, engaged in the pelvic motions, felt no pain or discomfort, and most conceived and became perfectly good mothers as well as wives. Except for this lack of desire, they may have even been the ideal wives. These are the cases where we hear the woman saying: "Sex? I can take it or leave it." She has no aversion to sex, but no desire or real interest in her human capacity for eroticism.

In some cases, this lack of desire is what we call "situational." This is most often found in the woman who professes to have no real desire for sex, yet can respond and even have an orgasm upon stimulation. If the husband initiates the sex, she is responsive, but if he doesn't she will be just as content. We call this case "situational" because some outside factor is interfering with the innate desire for sex. If this situation were altered to remove the intruding factor, she would more readily perceive that she does indeed have a desire for sex, perhaps even a very strong desire. One fairly common cause of this situation is an unrecognized anger that the woman may have for the husband and that she takes to bed with her. That serves as a kind of "Colonial Bundling Board" to keep the husband away. If the husband does not take the initiative and leap over this figurative board, they would never have sex. If you took the same woman and put her into bed with Lady Chatterly's lover (or the man of her erotic dreams), she would be an aggressive tigress. If you are that potential tigress, think about what you may be bringing to bed with you before you accept the belief that you have a very low libido.

There are many other kinds of situations that may result in lowered or even blocked libido, sexual desire or performance. In Chapters 4 through 7 we talk about these, and suggest ways you may possibly overcome them. Some of these are:

- *Stress from work, parenting, money shortages, etc.*
- *Fear of becoming pregnant*
- *Lack of erotic and sensual practice*—Not enough practice in pleasuring the body
- *Fear of sexual fantasizing, and revealing the subconscious*—Homosexual, incestuous, and other forbidden images come to mind
- *Problems with your partner*—Poor hygiene, weight gain, sexual illiteracy, anger

- *Medications, alcohol, and other drugs*—Over the counter medications like cold preparations, excessive drinking, opiates, "downers," and others
- *Changing male and female roles*—Coping with the more assertive woman, equality in marriage, and the elimination of the double standard
- *Aversion to genitalia*—Unconscious thoughts about the vagina or penis being "dirty," "smelly," or dangerous
- *Sexual abuse as a child or adult*—Incest, rape, sexual molestation, or psycho-sexual abuse
- *Poor self-image*—Growing up with verbal abuse by parents—"We hope you will be lucky enough to find some man who will marry you."
- *Boredom*—You've done it all: "Is that all there is, my friend?"

Now, let us make clear that it is not a case of either you do or you don't have desire. It is a matter of degree. Look at it as a scale of one to ten. How can we measure if you are a ten or an eight or a one? We can't! It's only a relative indicator that you can try to measure by how often and how intensely you think about sex and act upon those thoughts. We don't believe that there are people who have *no* desire for sex. There are those that have developed a negative desire—something that therapy could turn around to provide the person with the potential for a satisfying sex life. The first thing for such people is the recognition that their lack of sexual desire is something they probably have control over.

Can you move up your sexual desire quotient from a three to a seven? We believe you can, and we will discuss in subsequent chapters how you can heighten your desires by developing more erotic attitudes along with healthy self-esteem. Sexual desire may also go down several notches for some people. They may consciously lower their erotic profile if they are in a high-risk career or social situation in which it would be very risky if they allowed their sexual desires to get out of control. In some cases, women's sexual desire may fluctuate with hormonal influences during the menstrual phases.

To make matters more complicated, people vary in their desire for *variety* in sexual activity. Some people with a low desire for sex may still have a high desire for variety, while others with a very high desire for sex may be very much monogamous and monotonous in bed. Sex is never simple to understand! Ultimately, you have to evaluate your own desires and their impact on your love life. You'll know if you want to make it better.

CHAPTER 3

Men: What Are Your *Problems?*

When we were growing up in the 1940s, the sex manuals of the day, such as Van DeVelde's *Ideal Marriage,* were often very romantic and traditional. But, they usually presented a picture of sexuality in which the male had to curb his aggressive sexual appetite while slowly and lovingly engaging in foreplay with his essentially passive wife. His job was to "bring her" to a level of excitement whereby, after beginning coitus, he could skillfully time his movements so that the Great Moment of Climax occurred for them simultaneously. Trying not to come before she did, he had to "work" at increasing foreplay or else delay his ejaculation substituting passion with visions of filling out income tax returns. Yes, "Those were the days, my friend" when sex for the considerate male was construed as learning how to ignore his own passion.

Of course, times have changed and men are hopefully a little more sophisticated about the nature of female arousal and how to help a woman reach an orgasm—without resorting to mental gymnastics. But many men still have difficulties with timing their ejaculation or maintaining an erection during a passionate sexual encounter. Today, men can have it both: enjoying their own passion as well as their partner's, and being able to control the timing of their ejaculation. Later in Chapter 8 we will suggest the techniques for learning how to do this and maintaining an erection, but first let us examine the different kinds of problems that men often complain about.

For the most part, we can classify male sexual dysfunction difficulties into four main categories:

- Premature ejaculation
- Erectile difficulties
- Retarded ejaculation
- Lack of sexual interest

Note that "lack of sexual interest" is the only major complaint shared by both the men and the women who come to us for help. The causes for the problem are often the same, but, in some instances, they are also quite different.

Premature Ejaculation

This is not an easy situation to define because it means different things to different people. It is probably easiest to look at it from the broadest perspective. It is any ejaculation situation in which the male is dissatisfied with his timing—that is, it occurs too soon for him.

Too soon can mean many things:

- He gets so excited when making love that he ejaculates even before he can penetrate.
- He may ejaculate just as he is attempting penetration.
- He may ejaculate seconds after penetration even though he does not move.
- He may penetrate, begin thrusting, and ejaculate after very few movements.
- He may be thrusting in and out for many minutes and, even though he does not want to come so soon, his reflex actions produce an ejaculation.

Notice that what is common to all of these scenarios is that the man is not in control over *when* the ejaculation takes place. His body is in control, not his will. In other words, he is not satisfied with *when* his ejaculation occurs and it matters not whether it's before, during, or after penetration—even many minutes after—as long as the timing was not of his choosing.

Premature ejaculation may be considered the opposite problem of retarded ejaculation, when a man can not achieve orgasm within a reasonable time after he decides to. While some may think that this prolonged intercourse is desirable, we shall see that retarded ejaculation often results in the frustrating situation of no ejaculation at all. And certainly, the frustration that can result is very upsetting. While some of you may be thinking, "My husband should have such a problem," this is no laughing matter for many men.

Erectile Difficulties

How long should it take before a man develops a firm erection once he is being stimulated by his partner's touch? Should a man always get an erection by just thinking about a sexy person or sexy scene? How long should a man be able to maintain an erection while he is engaged in foreplay? And what about maintaining the erection after penetration and movement? Shouldn't a man get an erection when just kissing his lover? How hard should his erection be? Can a man have an erection while he is asleep but not when awake?

We get questions like this very often in calls to the Dr. Ruth shows and in letters to our columns. Our answers are necessarily less than specific because, as with premature ejaculation, erectile difficulties may be highly subjective. Basically, as long as a man is concerned about the hardness, frequency, or duration of his erection, he has a problem that is real to him. Whether the problem is due to a different physiological problem that now affects the erection, to some psychological factors, or merely to sexual illiteracy must be determined separately in each individual case. And our consideration must be based upon a good deal more information than mere dissatisfaction. Since this problem could possibly indicate a serious medical difficulty, we always err on the side of caution and say that one should rule out the physiological problems first. Before working on any possible psychological or situational causes with sex therapists, or even following our suggestions in the later chapters of this book, we recommend getting a clean bill of health from your family physician or urologist. Make sure that you tell your physician all the sexual symptoms and details of your problem.

Men are often the victims of a Catch-22 situation when it comes to their erectile difficulties. You see, they are worried that they may have a problem because they are not performing satisfactorily (at least not up to their own standards). Then, the stress this worry produces may cause them to perform poorly because stress is often the cause of erectile problems in many men. In other words, the concern that they *may* have some difficulties with an erection can actually *cause* the difficulty. This is sometimes called a "self-fulfilling prophecy" or "anticipatory anxiety." It seems that so many people are always fighting with themselves, doesn't it?

Now, there are different kinds of situations that may lead some men to think that they have a problem with their erections:

- The weakening of visual stimulation—that is, no longer getting erect from seeing nude women, viewing suggestive photos, or watching erotic movies.

- The weakening of physical stimulation—that is, no longer obtaining an erection from either self-stimulation or physical stimulation by others.
- A firm erection takes much more time and effort than it used to.
- An erection requires far more exotic kinds of stimulation—either in fantasy or in behavior—than before.

There are some men who report that they "never" get an erection and that they must be "sexless" or "impotent." These are two words we wish would disappear, because they are more misleading and frightening than they are useful in communication. Those men with great difficulties obtaining an erection—or having none at all—may have a physiological problem requiring a urologist. In some cases it may be due to medications taken for other reasons. If you are taking medications and you experience an erectile difficulty or loss of libido, your physician should be consulted. But, in many cases, there is really a situational factor that inhibits the erection. This is especially so for those men who are perfectly capable of having a fullblown hard erection while asleep. To argue that this is not a real erection because it is stimulated by bladder pressure or something else, is nonsense. As long as the apparatus works, the man is probably just as capable of having his erection in a sexual situation.

If you want a simple, but not necessarily foolproof, test to see if you *do* have erections in your sleep, take the "stamp test." Buy a roll of postage stamps from the post office. When you are ready to retire, take about 5 to 8 stamps in a strip and run it snugly around the base of your penis. Place a little moisture on the end of the last stamp so that they will stay in place during the night. Go to sleep and have pleasant dreams. If the strip of stamps is split when you get up in the morning, you probably had a good stiff erection. If it isn't, try again the next night, but make them a little snugger. Even though you think you don't have erections, you will probably find that you did during the night. If your apparatus is working (verify with the physician if you wish) then let's get down to working on the exercises in the rest of this book.

Now, let us look at those men who are able to obtain erections, but the erection is not as strong, as rigid, and as longlasting as it once was. The problem may tie in with:

- the diminished effect of visual stimulation
- the diminished effect of physical stimulation
- the longer time it takes to achieve an erection
- the need to use more exotic stimulation to attain even a soft erection.

A third class of erectile difficulties involves an all-too-brief erection before ejaculation. That is, the man complains that his penis gets soft before he has his climax, and that the orgasm occurs during the period in which his erection is waning. This man achieved an erection and a climax, but he begins to worry that he may run out of "hardness" in the future. Again, as in other difficulties, stress and worry are the real culprits. Learning how to "relax and enjoy it" are of vital importance.

Retarded Ejaculation

Many a sexually inexperienced man thinks that the only way he can truly satisfy a woman is for his penis to be thrusting in and out of her until she reaches orgasm. (See Chapter 9 to understand how harmful this kind of thinking may be for both the man and woman.) If, unfortunately, you ever held the erroneous view that the sensual beauty and pleasure of the sex act was merely like the pumping of pistons in a car's engine, then you might also have thought: "Hmm, the longer I can keep at it the more likely the woman is to climax; why can't I be as lucky as those men who can go on and on for hours without coming?"

First of all, they probably can't "go for hours"—it is usually empty bragging. Secondly, if they could, their poor partners would probably be hurting and not enjoying themselves at all. And most importantly, don't envy men who seem to have great staying power. Most of them would desperately like to achieve a climax within a reasonable amount of time—but they may not be able to climax when they want to. They may suffer from what is called "retarded ejaculation."

This is not an enviable condition. It involves both physical and emotional frustration, discomfort, and loss of interest. These men may experience anger, and they may question their own masculinity or sexual orientation. What some men do, therefore, is to turn a disturbing problem into a virtue. By bragging about staying power they can more easily avoid facing their problem while scoring some macho points with their friends. Some men even "advertise" to their women acquaintances that they don't come quickly because they are great lovers. But sadly, all of this may be a cover for a deeply rooted psychological problem.

For example, one young man we know of is very versatile in his lovemaking ability. Luckily, he has recently found a woman partner who is also very versatile and willing to vary her lovemaking techniques. The sad part of their wild lovemaking sessions is that although he is able to bring her to orgasm many times through oral sex as well as coitus, it seems that no matter how long he engages in coitus or no matter how long she fellates him, he has to help himself ejaculate through masturbation—either while the tip of his penis is in her mouth or by pulling out during coitus and masturbating over her body. At the beginning of therapy, he believed that he had to do this because his partner was too tired to continue fellatio or that he was too tired to continue coitus. The fact that he almost always had to masturbate in order to climax was somehow lost on him.

What this young man did not understand was that there was a deeply rooted sense of hostility in him toward the kind of sex life he was having. In the back of his mind there was the belief, going back to the early days of his puberty, that the "proper" sex act should end with him ejaculating into an idealized wife and thus creating a new life with that one perfect act of love. But, consciously, he was aware that this "idealization" was far from his present sex life, which was really in the socially experimental stage involving different women. Since he had a very strong libido, he would have sex frequently but inwardly hated this loveless sex. He had to force himself to ejaculate to relieve the sexual tension at these encounters, but he could not enjoy an easy, spontaneous climax like most men. Other men who have come in for treatment of retarded ejaculation appear to unconsciously block their climax because they are unable to give of themselves to a woman—not even their seminal fluid.

Now, it is certainly true that there are some men (and you may learn to become one if you wish) who can choose to delay their ejaculation until their partner has had an orgasm. This is fine if that is what both partners want. But the key word here is "choose." Someone experiencing retarded ejaculation is just as sexually out of control as the premature ejaculator. In short, only honest discussion with your partner about when she would like you to climax, coupled with your own honest feelings about when you would like to ejaculate will insure maximum satisfaction all around. When you cannot perform as well as you planned you may have a problem with either premature or retarded ejaculation. Consultation with a sex therapist is in order if you are often disappointed with the timing of your ejaculation.

Lack of Sexual Desire

Two of the most destructive and enduring sexual myths are 1) that women have to have their sexual feelings "aroused" by men and 2) that all men are "naturally" sexually aggressive and subject to strong sexual desires. We have discussed the first myth in the last chapter, and now we would like to explode the second myth. While all women are born with the potential for strong sexual desires, it must be nurtured and developed for it to become a positive force in one's life. Similarly with men. So what about the old sex researchers' belief that males peak in their sexual interest during their late teens while many women don't peak until their forties or even fifties? What these sex experts overlooked was the role that culture played in helping the male nurture his sexual interest, while at the same time inhibiting the female from nurturing her sexual interest. What do we mean by this?

It is not uncommon for prepubescent boys to swap jokes about sex and pass pornographic pictures among one another or even to practice group "jerk-off" (masturbation) sessions to see who could ejaculate quickest or for younger boys to have the older boys demonstrate masturbation. The young boy's peer group is all very much interested in sex—knowledge of sexual activities, terms, techniques, and more are much admired and rewarded by the peer group. As we know from Kinsey and other researchers, masturbation is almost universal for boys around the time of puberty and during their adolescence. Thus they have many years of encouraged fantasy, visual erotic stimulation, and, most importantly, physical stimulation of the penis to the point of climax. This is all very important for the nurturance of the physiological response of stimulation-to-climax of the penis. As a result, most young men have little difficulty with arousal and climax. As the male gets older, however, becomes a father, and works harder and later hours at his job, the pressures of work cause undue stress. And we certainly know what impact stress may have on one's libido and sex life. So, the observation that male teenagers are wild and horny while a forty-five year old man would rather watch TV and have a few beers may have some truth to it, but now we can suspect situational factors rather than hormones alone.

When we compare the psycho-sexual development of girls in our culture, we see just the opposite of the male pattern. Especially, in the past, the subculture of the prepubescent and early adolescent girl did not show any obsession with, or even much interest in, sex—not because the potential was absent, but because there was no reward from her peers for sexual precociousness. Masturbation was not encouraged by peers. While some girls secretly did masturbate, we know that guilt often developed due to the prevailing attitudes that a girl should not touch herself "down there." While this was also told to boys, the boys had a peer group to negate that message; the girls did not.

By the time they got married the orgasmic reflex system of many young women in the past, had little, if any, exercising. Their husbands, on the contrary, had 10 years or more of "nurturing." No wonder so many women complained that their husbands always wanted to have sex while men complained just the opposite about their wives. As the marriage progressed, however, the pressures of work took their toll on the male and the increasing stress affected their sex lives. The traditional woman, beginning her erotic life during the courtship period or just after marriage, experienced a delay in her erotic nurturance—but at least she was on her way to catching up with her husband. As the marriage progressed for the woman, the stresses she had to endure as homemaker and mother began to ease as the youngest children were finishing high school and leaving for college. Unfortunately, just at the time when she could most enjoy a sexual renaissance, the stress was probably highest for her husband.

This is why we say that culture, not nature, played a negative trick on the sexual libido of men and women who grew up before the sixties. But today, this is no longer the case. More young girls are nurturing their sexual libido and exercising their orgasmic-reflex system through masturbation as well as early sexual activity. That is the good news—at least for the libido, if not for the parent—but the bad news is that many women, are moving into the competitive labor force and are experiencing the same kinds of stresses that their husbands are. This has created new problems that we will address in Chapter 7.

Understanding the role of culture helps us more clearly define the problems a male might have with sexual desire. For example, a male might reach manhood, take on a wife, father some children, and soon find himself having little sexual desire or interest. This does not mean that he doesn't love his wife, that he is latently homosexual, or some other simplistic explanation. We are talking about the type of lack of desire where it makes no difference who the partner is. Although he may appear to be bored with his wife, he's not even ripe for an extra-marital affair. In some cases, weeks or months may pass by in their marriage before the husband and wife engage in any sexual activity. His wife may have wanted sex, but she might feel uncomfortable about initiating sex due to his apparent loss of interest. He might even feel that he should have sex, but the desire is too weak to motivate him.

We are not referring to situations where loss of desire has resulted from a change in the relationship, but rather where there is still love but no desire. In some cases, he may never have been moved by much "horniness" or physical desire, while in others there is a marked loss of desire over the years. We have seen cases where a recent operation or a touch of heart trouble elicited enough fear to drive a husband's desire away. In one case, a man had one testicle that had not descended and another testicle that did not develop properly. He was perfectly capable of having sex, but he believed that no woman could be interested in him. Shame and self-doubt just pushed sex out of his mind. This is similar to a women who may lose sexual interest after a mastectomy or some other operation. She puts it into her mind that she couldn't be attractive, so she defensively avoids intimacy and the possibility of rejection.

We know that these men and women are not sexually dead. These same men and woman can show an interest in sex—reading steamy novels, watching erotic movies, talking or thinking about it—but yet they have no real desire to initiate and complete a sexual act. That is, they are lacking "horniness"—that sense of urgency to have sex.

Sometimes, men (and women) may have such strong negative images or even disgust about the sex organs that they don't like to think about sex. They feel, or have been taught, that the sex organs are dirty, that they are somehow dangerous, or the tools of the Devil's temptations. They might even have an irrational fear that somehow the vagina may injure the penis. Now, when a person does not want to think about sex at all, when he can not comfortably hear about it, talk about it or do anything about it, this is probably a deeply rooted problem for the psychotherapist who must try to uncover these severe emotional blocks against sex. The sex therapist can only help to suggest if this course of action is needed, but will not usually attempt to directly treat strong psychological blocks without coordinated help from other therapists. If you have the less severe problems of lost sexual desire we will discuss later in Chapters 8 and 9 the steps you may take to resolve these problems.

There are other concerns men have that are not as disturbing as not being able to achieve an erection or loss of desire. Just as worrisome to some men, however, is the length of time before the urge to have sex returns to the sexually active man. The post-ejaculation recovery time is an important part of a man's feelings about his vigor and sexuality.

This recovery time is what we call the refractory period, and it has to do with both psychological situations and the ability of the body to regenerate the seminal fluids for the ejaculation. Some delays in recovery time may be situational—and these we will discuss in Chapters 8 and 9. Otherwise, the longer refractory period may only follow the natural process of getting a little older. In this case, we have to learn to become a little more creative and imaginative to help nature along. But remember, the normal refractory period is different with each man. For some it may be hours, but for others it may be days. For a few, usually when they are fairly young, it may even be minutes. In any case, if the man is concerned by the length of recovery time, there are ways of shortening the time period.

Other Problems

There is still another kind of male problem that has to do with the perceived strength and intensity of the orgasm. The man says that, it just doesn't feel as good as it once did. He may not be able to adequately express what the difference is, but he knows that the force and his own pleasure during ejaculation has somewhat diminished. This is a very subjective problem, because, as with any other experience involving the appreciation of a sensory or sensual experience, it greatly depends on one's setting, the expectations, the mood, the partner, the man's overall health conditions, and a whole host of other situational and extraneous factors. A perceived loss of intensity in the orgasmic response may also be found among some women. These situational disappointments are usually overcome by creating the ideal conditions that the individuals believe will produce the most satisfying orgasms. More on this later.

Some men report that they have difficulties with erections because they feel some pain when attaining the erection, when they ejaculate, or when they have intercourse. Sometimes such pain is restricted to female-superior sexual positions or to other specific sexual activities. In all these cases we strongly urge the man to see a urologist to check out the causes of the pain.

Overcoming the Myths

All too often there are sexual myths, rather than real sexual problems, that give some men causes for anxiety. For example, there is often concern about the amount of ejaculate becoming less over time. While there may be some pathological condition causing this (and if you are concerned, consult with your urologist), for most men this merely reflects the natural diminution due to getting a little older. The belief that the amount of ejaculate somehow reflects a man's potency is the result of the macho myth that a man must have an ejaculate the size of a bull's! Indeed, there are sexually illiterate men who strongly believe that the quantity of their ejaculate is a reflection on their masculinity, that a quarter of a cup indicates a sexual "Superman" while a tablespoon points to a "wimp." Such nonsense! The seminal fluid is merely the vehicle for the semen to be discharged into the vaginal canal so that the little sperm swimmers can begin their journey.

Masculinity is a matter of social quality, not physical quantity. Among other things, real masculinity has to do with how a male relates to a woman: how considerate he is, how loving he is, how well he excites and pleases her, and how sensitive he is to her emotional and physical needs. The worth of a man as a lover or life partner can not be measured in tablespoons of ejaculate nor in inches of erect penis!

This macho myth concerning the quantity of the ejaculate has another side to it. There are men who worry because, as they get a little older, the force of the ejaculation grows less. Instead of spurting out a few inches or more, they complain that the semen only trickles out. While this may be due to some physical problems—again, check it out with your urologist—for most men, it is no indication of any problem whatsoever. It certainly has nothing to do with how great a lover you are or if you are able to father more children. The quality of a man's orgasms and love life depends on the sexiness of his mind, not the force and volume of his seminal fluids. An eighty-year-old man can have a good, loving, active, satisfying sexual relationship, while a twenty-year-old with all the right quantitative advantages can have an unsatisfactory and loveless sex life.

Now, don't confuse semen trickling out during orgasm with "seepage"—that is, small amounts of seminal fluid that leak out when there is no sexual excitement involved and no nocturnal emission with an accompanying orgasm. Sometimes, without having contractions and an orgasm, the semen slowly trickles out without any great sensation. If this occurs, the man should see a urologist. This seepage should not be confused with a pre-ejaculatory drop of liquid, which may contain semen. This often appears during sexual excitement, and is a fairly common phenomenon. This drop is of no concern, but it does prove that the withdrawal tactic is a very poor method of contraception. If any one of these pre-ejaculatory drops contains spermatozoa, a man can impregnate a woman without an ejaculation.

Sometimes a seepage of semen occurs with either the straining accompanying a bowel movement or during urination. These may be very natural, indicating that the man has not had an ejaculation for some time. However, for a few, this may indicate a urological condition. If this happens to you on more than rare occasions, you should consult with your urologist. What? You have no urologist? No excuses! Just as every woman needs a gynecologist to see regularly, to ensure the well-being of that very important area of her body, every man should have a urologist that he can comfortably consult for any problems that might arise. We find that many men delay seeing a physician about sexual or genital problems because they are uncomfortable talking about these issues. Don't you be one of them! Your health and your genitalia deserve more respect than that!

Painful Testicles

And then, there are "blue balls"—which almost every teenage boy knows about, but sometimes forgets as an adult. This is a painful condition involving the penis and testicles due to repeated and prolonged sexual excitation without subsequent ejaculation. When long-term blood engorgement in this area builds up without orgasmic relief there can be much discomfort or pain. (Women have something similar to this, but there is no popular term for it. Perhaps something like "blue lips" should enter the vocabulary.) Sometimes, adult men get "blue balls" when they get sexually aroused for a period of time but do not have a partner to help satisfy their needs. The solution for this condition is simple: You need to have sex with someone or to masturbate. If you can not or will not ejaculate by having sex or masturbating (perhaps because of religious reasons), then you must avoid sexual stimulation. There are no silly solutions like taking a cold shower or running around the block. The bodies of men and women are designed to have sex—without our sexual instincts and needs the human race would die out. We were meant to have sex. Let's do nature's bidding in the healthiest, most ethically responsible, loving and satisfying manner that we can!

CHAPTER 4

Relax and Enjoy: Stress-Reduction Techniques

Before we can recommend specific ways to overcome one or more of the problems we mentioned in the last two chapters, it is important to develop the skills to create the right conditions and environment both within yourself and in your surroundings. We are referring to skills that many people like yourself *need* to help pave the way for fulfilling sex. In fact, these skills are of help to all of us in our daily activities—at work, at home, and at play—and are not merely applicable and effective in overcoming sexual difficulties.

Many health professionals believe that among the most important skills that all human beings need are different ways of reducing stress. Before many people can *begin* to develop a control over their sexual problems, they must first learn to control the problems of stress. Why? Because, good sex doesn't mix with stress, tension, and anxiety.

We have to learn different kinds of relaxation techniques for different kinds of situations. We need to develop techniques of social relaxation, that is, learning to control certain environmental factors that might cause us stress; aesthetic relaxation, such as creating a mood and physical setting conducive to relaxation (you know, candles, music, wine, etc.); and physical relaxation techniques. These physical techniques can help many people reduce the stress that is interfering with the spontaneous reflex action in male and female orgasm. For men, this stress or anxiety may either inhibit the orgasmic response, or it can even cause premature ejaculation—two problems just taken up in Chapter 3. Ejaculation before penetration or soon after is usually related to nervousness—the layman's phrase for stress-induced anxiety.

During the past ten years or so, many physicians and psychologists have done a lot of research on the impact of stress on one's life. On the level of physical health we know that unless a person is able to reduce or cope with a good deal of everyday stress that person may be subject to ulcers, heart trouble, high blood pressure, and a host of other physical problems. It seems that every day we learn more and more about the harmful effects of stress on the body. On the psychological level, it appears that stress may interfere with normal emotional and libidinal functioning. For most people, there appears to be no doubt that stress can be a complete turn-off, an inhibitor of sexual arousal, sexual feelings, and sensuous pleasures.

We believe that stress may be blamed in many cases, for what may appear to be a sexual dysfunction or a problem of sexual dissatisfaction. Before you get involved in the exercises that we suggest later in this book, you must get to know yourself and determine whether stress is blocking your ability to relax.

Now, just what do we mean by stress? The person who made a major impact in the medical profession in this area was the great physician Hans Selye, who died just a few years ago. What he learned is that all human beings, just like other animals, react with what he called a "flight or fight syndrome" when they learn that they are in danger. Something could actually be threatening their physical existence, or, in the case of sensitive humans, threatening their psychological or social well-being—even their self-image. Selye noted and measured all the things that happen to our bodies when we believe that we are in some kind of danger: Our hearts beat faster, some of the muscles tense up, the pupils of the eye may dilate, blood pressure goes up, breathing comes faster and more shallow, we may break out in sudden cold sweat, the adrenaline pumps faster, and so forth. Nature, in this way, is gearing up the body to fight off that which is threatening us or to enable us to run as fast as we can away from the danger—fight or flight. The human body inherited this survival mechanism from mankind's earliest days.

Selye and other researchers of this "flight or fight syndrome" tell us that once we knew that we were safe, this syndrome was "turned off" and our bodily functions returned to normal. But today, in our more civilized world, things are more complex. Today, we are not dodging dinosaurs or battling saber-toothed tigers but confronting social, psychological, and economic fears. We worry about losing our jobs, not having enough money, getting older, what the neighbors think about our six-year-old-car, whether we are still man or woman enough to keep our spouse from straying—and more. Some people are afraid of walking from their cars to their homes at night, while others worry about international tensions. Compared to the physical dangers facing a Stone Age hunter these trials may seem trivial, but we modern corporate battlers and income gatherers get just as "fearful" or "anxious" or "nervous" or "uncomfortable"—synonyms for the gut reaction we feel when the flight or fight syndrome is turned on in our bodies—when we merely face emotional or psychological danger, even to our self-esteem. Our worries are as real and stressful to us as physical dangers would be. But, if you perceive that your boss is threatening your livelihood by firing you, you can't kill your boss—and you can't always quit when you want to. If your ego is threatened because your wife or husband is no longer crazy about you, your civilized training and religious beliefs and concern for the children may not permit you to even separate. Yet, you must learn to control the impact of stress upon you. Now, if we don't turn off this protective mechanism by getting rid of the source of the stress, or learning to manage stress, that tension will stay with us. And—for our considerations in this book—the consequence of this stress is to fill us with worries and anxieties that hamper our ability to have a good sexual experience.

So, what do we do about the stress that we bring to bed? It is not always easy to remove the source of the stress. We can't always guarantee ourselves job security or a well-padded bank account, and we can't prevent the aging process. We can't always keep up with the Joneses and we can't lock up our straying spouse. Fortunately, there is a way to reduce the end result of this stress. It involves a skill that we all have within us, which can be activated in one manner or another.

It was another great physician, Herbert Benson, who elaborated upon the mechanism that enables us to turn off the "flight or fight syndrome." He believed that we'd suffer much physical and psychological harm if we don't. He reasoned that if nature was so ingenious as to give us this flight or fight syndrome that protects us by temporarily increasing our muscular strength and mental readiness to run or fight, then nature must have also provided for a means to turn off this syndrome at will.

Dr. Benson identified a physiological control mechanism, which we already have within us, to enable us to deal with stress on a very personal and safe level. He called this the "relaxation response" and described it in his book of the same name. He said that there are many ways that a person can turn off the stress through relaxation techniques such as engaging in various athletic activities, controlled breathing, meditation, or prayer. But he suggests that the easiest and least intrusive way to turn off the "fight or flight syndrome" is through the "relaxation response." He also knew that reducing stress through the "relaxation response" can help stressed-out people to regain their ability to have good sex.

In the area of sex, the problem of stress is particularly acute because people sometimes create their own sexual performance anxiety. A man may worry to himself, "am I going to be able to keep up my erection," and a woman might worry, "am I going to please him enough to satisfy him." *Because* of this stress they both don't do well—their sexual anxiety becomes a self-fulfilling prophecy. We find that many people who have sexual problems have these negative scenarios, these anxieties, in their heads when they approach sex, and that we must help them get over this negative thinking.

But what are some of the things you might do on your own to reduce non-sexual stress that crawls in bed with you? Well, first, there is the technique that Dr. Benson recommends in his books. It is a simple meditative exercise, done twice a day for twenty minutes each time. Essentially, it boils down to sitting in a quiet, comfortable place where you will not be disturbed, closing your eyes, becoming conscious of your breathing, and saying to yourself the number one with each exhalation. After a while you will not think about anything else. If you do, you again repeat the number one to yourself until that is all you see in your mind. The objective is to clear the head of all "chatter"—the nagging, gnawing thoughts that are a source of stress for many of us—for about 20 minutes. We know it sounds too simple to be true, but many who have performed this exercise and other forms of meditation have been helped in many areas of their lives where problems have resulted in part due to stress—including physical problems.

Ask your physician about this technique, because more and more physicians are urging people to learn these stress-reducing techniques. He or she may be able to refer you to a place near your home where you will learn much more about these simple, safe, and effective meditation exercises.

Now other people prefer more physical means of closing out stressful thoughts. These tend to be athletic activities that push people to the limits of their physical abilities: skiing, tennis, mountain climbing, racquetball, handball, running, and so forth. We are not all in agreement as to why these reduce stress, but many of them do work for many people. Some people say it is because it releases a chemical in the brain that calms us down, others say it is because it gives us enhanced self-esteem and self-confidence. Still others say that it is because of the intense concentration you need to perform well at higher levels of athletic skills, and that this concentration is like the meditation in the "relaxation response" that closes off stressful chatter.

While you are intensely concentrating about a physical activity you cannot think about that professional deadline, about family problems, and so forth. It doesn't seem to work in more simple exercising, such as walking, because when you walk you often think about your problems even more because you have very little else to do. (However, if you do what is called "power" or "speed" walking, which requires a great deal of concentration, it can help to reduce stress in the manner we have described.) It also doesn't work in entertaining activities such as watching TV or going to the movies. These are often opportunities to identify with characters who are going through stress and to be reminded of your own anxieties. Even fishing, which epitomizes relaxing activity for many people, too often allows the mind to wander to stress-inducing thoughts and memories, while you are waiting for the fish to nibble at your bait.

You want to create a situation in which you have this "20 minutes of nothingness" in your brain on a regular basis at least once or twice a day. During this "20 minutes of nothingness" you fool the brain into turning off whatever degree of the "flight or fight syndrome" is present by making the brain believe everything is peaceful—that there are no psychological or social threats to our self-esteem or well-being.

For some people, meditation or the "relaxation response" techniques of Benson won't work because these just don't fit their personalities—they feel funny doing them. For others, strenuous athletics may not be suitable for health or other reasons. Fortunately, there are many other simple things that people may do to reduce stress, depending upon their interests and inclinations:

Prayer

Go to a quiet place in your church or synagogue and, with your eyes closed, repeatedly recite a one-line prayer in your mind for about twenty minutes. Allow the prayer to take over your consciousness so that you are no longer thinking about saying the prayer but it seems to flow into your mind of its own accord.

Music

In a quiet relaxed setting in your home, listen to a very familiar and beloved piece of restful music with your eyes closed. Imagine that you and the music are one. Do not think about the music; feel its presence inside you until you are soaring with the melody. We find that what is called *charismatic* music—such as Gregorian chants, Hassidic music, church organ music, or Gospel music—works well with many people.

Poetry

Listen with your eyes closed, in a private, quiet setting, to a record of poetry readings that you know well and love to hear. Don't try to think of what the poet means by this or that phrase or word. Allow the imagery to go past your conscious mind so that you feel the poetry as if you and the poet are one. Isn't it amazing how few people still read or listen to poetry? It is the music of words. For many people it can provide an experience of serenity like nothing else. Try it, you'll like it!

Environmental sounds

Go to a conducive setting, listening to a record of the sounds of rain, of the wind, or of the surf crashing on the beach. These records are readily available at any record shop or they can be ordered for you if they are not in stock. Listen to these sounds in the same manner as we recommended for music and poetry. Don't use them as a background for your thoughts but instead, try to suspend your thinking and just visualize that you are in a most beautiful place by yourself, with these sounds reinforcing the beauty of your imagined situation. Concentrate on the sounds until you forget your body and thoughts. Again, let your body become one with the sounds.

Dancing

Patterned dancing in which people whirl around can also reduce stress, such as American square dancing, European circle dances of all kinds, and practically all forms of folk dancing. Some writers, such as the physician Andrew Weil, believe that many dances, particularly ones where people spin around and around, may, just as meditation can do, meet an inborn need to "alter consciousness" and are the adult version of the spinning we see in children throughout the world. An interesting notion—but no matter what the explanation, this dizzying kind of dancing seems to reduce stress for many people. Although more formal and requiring more training, ballet dancing is another good form of stress reduction.

Sailing

When you have reached a level of knowledge where you no longer have to think about what you are doing but can become one with the water and wind and sun and boat and sail, you can experience a sense of peace and relaxation beyond words. It can be what the psychologist Abraham Maslow called a peak experience—one which elevates you beyond the normal day-to-day living experiences. Albert Einstein used sailing as the antithesis of the intellectual world he lived in—sailing was for him a world that becomes physical and spiritual at the same time. It is interesting that many people have said that when sex is best it is because, through love, the partners have created an environment in which it, too, is physical and spiritual at the same time.

A word here about what not to do. With the exception perhaps of a glass or two of wine before or with dinner, alcohol and other drugs do not really make us relax by turning off the "flight or fight syndrome." They don't reduce stress. They merely deceive the thinking part of the brain, that is your awareness, into believing that everything is more peaceful, better, less dangerous, etc. The stress that was there before still remains, but when you drink to excess and want to try to reduce stress through the means we suggest above, it won't work. You cannot get the benefits that you would from meditation or prayer or music or athletics or any other nonchemical means of reducing stress when you have alcohol in your bloodstream.

We have another suggestion for you. Since the focus of this book is on helping you overcome sexual difficulties and enhancing your sexual skills, we think it would be a good idea if you could learn one or more of these stress-reducing techniques *with a partner.* The reason for this is to learn how to do something important and pleasurable with someone else—an activity that, when it is performed correctly, is not dependent on conscious thought as much as a sort of *feeling* of the experience. We think that this is a good idea, because too many of the bad sexual experiences people have are based upon intellectualizing, thinking, worrying, projecting one's thought onto the other, and so forth.

There are times, such as in a good, loving, sexual experience where you want to just do and feel without intruding your intellect into the situation. It's good to get into the habit of doing this, with your partner, in other areas, so it can carry over into your sex life. There's no sweeter mantra than "I love you" or "We are one."

Romance

What most people forget, it seems, is that good old romance is one of the oldest means of reducing stress related to a sexual encounter. As the concept of romance and romantic love developed out of the Medieval period in our history, it meant the *idealization* of a situation. People then abstracted an essence from poetry, from music, from art that was pure, that didn't have all the unnecessary and often negative images or "chatter" that detract from beauty. So in romantic thinking, one saw only the beauty in someone. You forgot about the blemishes, the wrinkle, the spare tire at the midriff, and so forth. Thus, you concentrate only on the essence of the person, related to his or her beauty as a person. As Dr. Helen Singer Kaplan has said: When your husband comes home, you are not likely to be successfully aroused if you concentrate on his balding hair or his pot belly. But too frequently, many people do exactly that. They may be somewhat aroused during the day, and would like to have sex with their husbands or wives, but when they see their spouses at home and concentrate on the negative, their desire flies out the window. People have to concentrate on the positive aspects of the other person and to set up romantic *conditions* that will enhance desire rather than defeat it.

For example, the woman or man, could take a *bubble bath by candlelight* while the partner helps in the bathing by rubbing the back, providing a sip of wine, or reading some romantic poetry. Then they could switch places. Sounds corny—but romantic! If you can't do it because of children at home, try it in a hotel once in a while or send the kids over to the grandparents for the evening. Of course, you have to plan for such events, but lack of spontaneity won't detract from the fun and benefit it will be for both of you. Sex is such an important part of marital happiness that you must make the time for it. After all, what is more important, sex or going bowling? Don't answer that!

Bathing, aside from cleanliness, has other romantic implications for our thinking. It seems that more and more people take showers rather than baths. Why? Because people today are so much more on the move. A shower is conducive to getting in, getting cleaned, and getting out—a functional act without any real sensuous experience for most. Maybe it's an imperfect analogy, but it seems to us that it is reminiscent of the "Wham, bam, thank-you-ma'am" sort of sex that men have been criticized for. Both acts are similar in that need takes precedence over the possible sensuous experiences of a longer activity.

We believe that people should luxuriate more in the sensuous pleasures of their own bodies. Even when you are alone, take a bubble bath and use bath oils. Listen to soft music while you soak in the tub and think pleasant thoughts. You will learn to create a mood of romantic anticipation the more you do this during the week. Wash yourself slowly and feel the sensations as your hands touch each and every part of your body in a sensual and loving manner. We don't believe that this is a trivial and foolish activity for anyone of any age. We do believe that, on the contrary, it is conducive to feeling good about yourself, to developing a more positive self-image. It is even good for your physical and mental health. Why do we say this? It is because we believe that taking a long, sensual bath is like a bridge between the reality of the world, which can be very stressful, and what you are trying to achieve by way of a good sexual relationship in bed—which cannot be accomplished without reducing stress. In between the real external world and your bedroom you have to learn to reduce or control stress so that you don't take it to bed with you. It may take a bag of tricks to do this, but any romantic act that also reduces stress can be useful.

Eyeballing

Another good exercise that is stress reducing for most couples, and may even be erotically stimulating at the same time, is an old technique known as "eyeballing." To do this, sit fully dressed in comfortable chairs, facing your partner or spouse. With the lights low and some quiet music in the background, sit so that your knees are just touching and you are holding each other's hands. Make sure that each of your bodies are not sitting in a strained position. When you are quite comfortable, look into each other's eyes, *without saying a word* for about 20 minutes. You may blink, of course, but try to keep looking only into each other's eyes while holding hands. Remember, the eyes are the "windows to the soul," and each of you should experience some very pleasing, peaceful, intimate, and warm sensations flowing from you to your partner. Try it, it's fantastic!

Flower concentration

This is another thing you might try when you are alone. Get yourself a beautiful, fresh flower. Again, in that comfortable room where you will have some privacy, hold the flower in your hands and concentrate on the beauty of it for 15 to 20 minutes. Don't think about the beauty, feel it—feel the colors and the shades and the contours and the texture and the scent. If any outside thoughts come to mind, push them out with a concentration on the beauty of the flower you are looking at. Remember, you have the power to make a thought stop in this exercise as in others we have discussed. It may take some patience and practice, but isn't it worth it to achieve some of the peace you can get by reducing stress and some of the better sex you will have when you are a more relaxed person?

Sunshine

Perhaps the oldest and most common way to reduce stress is to get more in tune with nature. Long hikes in isolated areas, without the noise of the everyday world intruding, can be most relaxing. But unless you do it the right way, it can be counter-productive. If you just walk and allow your thoughts to flow wherever they want to, this stream of consciousness will frequently turn to thoughts of what is bothering you at home or at work. This is exactly what you want to avoid because this will be stress inducing rather than stress reducing. What you must do to use hiking as a stress-reduction technique is to concentrate, for longer and longer periods of time, on the natural beauty around you. You don't want to walk with your problems, you want to walk away from them. It is particularly useful to become knowledgeable about the flowers or the trees and look for and identify these as you walk along. This will help focus your thoughts on nature rather than yourself. Many people find that bird watching is an excellent way to reduce stress since it requires a great deal of concentration and focussed thinking to find and identify a bird through its song or flight or shape or plumage. And what can be more beautiful than a bird?

When in the world of nature, push the intrusive negative thoughts of the world of everyday reality right out of your mind. Many people find that being in a natural setting without any clothing on and feeling the breeze on the entire body is a most relaxing experience. Certainly, you must take precautions by blocking out the harmful sun rays if you burn easily, but sunbathing, even with a bathing suit on, can be very satisfying. To achieve the maximum stress-reduction benefit, this should be done in a quiet place with only loved ones nearby. We discussed nudist camps in our last book, *Sex and Morality*. We explained that the most important reason given for spending time in nudist camps is the strong sense of relaxation and stress reduction that accompanies swimming and sunbathing in the nude. If you might be so inclined, give it a try. It might work for you or it might not. But with or without bathing suits, sunlight seems to chase away many of our ordinary daily "blues."

In a sense, there are some strong psychological ramifications to what we are suggesting here. Instead of saying, "I can't help myself, this is the way I think and feel and I have no control over it," we must learn to say, "I have the ability to get rid of the negative and distracting thoughts that interfere with my life." It is so important to understand that we have within us the ability to control our own thoughts, behavior, and passions and not allow circumstances or emotions to overwhelm or control us. We know, for example, that two of the most serious problems in our society—alcoholism and narcotics addiction—are, in their most serious stages of progression, the result of loss of control when these substances are used or an inability to refrain from using them even when one wants to refrain. We need much practice to develop faith in ourselves as well as a spiritual life that can help us to change the destructive, negative thoughts and behavior in all areas of life.

Especially in the area of sex is this so important, because we do find stress, negative thoughts, and self-doubts intruding upon the marital relationship, upon the sexual relationship, and upon the spontaneous orgasmic reflex needed for a satisfying love life. In this chapter and those to follow we hope to help you get some control over parts of your life through these simple little exercises. It is important to have even small successes in learning how to push away even a trivial thought, like how bald your husband is becoming, when that thought is intruding upon your overall sexual desire for your husband. It is not sufficient for a critic to say: "That's such a superficial attitude. How could she let something so trivial affect her sexual feelings for her husband?" The fact is that women sometimes do feel this way, but they must learn how to push the feeling out of their minds so that they do not act upon these thoughts in a destructive manner. The more successful they become at controlling these trivial thoughts, the more able they will be at coping with the major stress-producing events.

Stress, like a virus, may be carried over to you by the friends and acquaintances who surround you. That is, their negativism and self-doubts due to *their own* stress become contagious when brought to you by these "friends." Because they are "down" people and very often pessimistic, they seem to contaminate and depress the people around them. If you confide in these friends that you would like to spice up your married sex life, they will tell you to "act your age." They want to make everyone around them as joyless as they are. Everyone knows such people. Be careful that you don't have too many of them around to drain you of energy and joy. If you have a friend who is always putting you down, drop that friend. With "friends" like these, who needs enemies? This doesn't mean that you should be insensitive to a friend's problems, but beware, if discussing problems—theirs or yours—seems to be the only "joy" of that person's life.

There is a special problem that we would like to address for a moment, and that is the problem of loneliness. This shadow could be cast upon your life due to widowhood, divorce, relocation to another city, or whatever. What is this topic doing in a chapter on stress reduction? It is because loneliness is almost certain to produce a great deal of stress for practically everybody. Humans need other humans to be around. It is not that people can't be *alone* if they want to. We can even enjoy being alone at times, but the special, good feelings that we all get when we are with people whom we love and who love us, and the intimacy of one-on-one relationships are not easy to give up. When circumstances change, over which we have no control, and we feel alone, even abandoned, stress is created that must be addressed. What can be done about it?

We believe that the *first step* is to examine your own particular circumstances and to determine that if you are lonely, you must understand that you have allowed yourself to become powerless in this area. It is no disgrace or shortcoming to be lonely but some people try to deny it and put up a happy front. Some even go so far as to rationalize that they are always happy when they are by themselves—even when deep down inside they know they are not. Once you recognize that you are lonely, you can make the right steps to change the situation. It is interesting to note that a recent study reported in *Modern Maturity* pointed out that older people who are widowed and who get pets to keep them company are more likely to remain healthy than those who live alone without pets. The reason given for this is that the owners are giving of themselves to their pets, giving love and care and nurturing just like they gave to their own children and spouses when they were younger. By giving and being concerned for their pets, they were less concerned and worried about themselves. In a sense, their stress is deflected and reduced in much the same way that we discussed earlier in this chapter with relaxation techniques. These pet owners had cut down on the negative chatter in their heads, and their more positive feelings emerged. Similarly, other activities that get lonely people out of their isolation and into active social gatherings can help reduce the stress that many feel from being alone, particularly when they are middle-aged or older.

Finally, let's discuss the oldest, and to many people the best, area of activities to help reduce stress: religion. It seems that in the last few decades people have increasingly minimalized the importance of religion in their lives. True, there are times and issues in which the mainstream religions seem to contradict in morals, ethics, and values what it is that their adherents sincerely believe and practice in their daily lives. We dealt with this subject extensively in our last book, *Sex and Morality*. But some disagreement with specific tenets or rituals doesn't mean that religion cannot still be a powerful force in our lives. Religion addresses the areas of anxiety and stress that result from those profound questions, doubts, and fears that all humans have by virtue of their mortality. Remember, it is religion and not science that deals with those questions beyond our comprehension—like death and the hereafter.

Religion doesn't have to be all or nothing. You can take control in your own religion, and make it more vital and meaningful to *you*. If you belong to a church or synagogue that doesn't seem to have enough activities and interests for you, take the initiative and devote some of your talent and energies to making it a better place for others, as well as yourself. The ritualized ceremonies, the repetition of familiar chants, melodies, and prayers, through times of joy and times of turmoil, add much-needed continuity through ritual that can be enormously satisfying to many people. Even nonbelievers find that they experience a sense of peace during the performance of these familiar rituals and ceremonies.

Some churches and synagogues have taken bold steps to provide a less stressful and more nurturing world for the congregants by creating artificial "extended" families of 25-50 persons who meet regularly together for dinners and celebrations. They also act as a support system to share grief as well as joy, providing intellectual stimulation and banishing loneliness. These groups can be very valuable in reducing stress for newcomers to a community or for anyone undergoing a crisis situation such as death or divorce. We believe that as the extended family becomes smaller and smaller—so much so that even the American nuclear family shrinks down to only *one* parent and children—people have to think of ways to provide substitute families for the millions of people who are geographically separated from their biological relatives. As many of our readers are well aware, being a single parent can be enormously stressful. We need more resources, both external and internal (like the ones at the beginning of this chapter), the better to enable people to handle stress.

In brief, while we cannot know if any particular sexual

problem is due to stress, it is important for you to understand the role of stress before concluding that a problem lies elsewhere. Even where there is no sexual dysfunction problem, the role of stress as an inhibitor of desired sexual response and pleasure is well known and accepted. So, no matter who you are, work on reducing stress to gain more control over your ability to think, feel, and act positively.

CHAPTER 5

Modern Technology and Sensual Pleasure

Some people may wonder why we would talk about mechanical and electronic gadgets as means to help us enjoy the very natural physiological and psychological responses of the sexual experience. Certainly, sex is a very natural activity, which is best when spontaneous and in a loving relationship with someone. But if sex were merely instinctual, there would be no need for this book and certainly no need for sex therapists. Unfortunately, human sexuality is more complex and therefore offers more possibilities for variation on a theme.

Many men and women, young and old, married and unmarried, need a little help to achieve spontaneous, natural, and satisfying sexual experiences and relationships. Just because one uses a mechanical or electronic device does not make something less natural. After all, on artificial electric and gas stoves we cook the most wonderful of sensual delights involving taste. We use complex mechanical and electronic instruments to create incredible sounds that are pleasing to the ear. We use mechanical and electronic complexities of state-of-the-art camera and sound equipment to create movies that can even be intellectually and emotionally overpowering as well as visually stunning. So, you see, it is not mechanical or electronic gadgets that count, but rather the very human and very natural results that are being enhanced.

We don't suggest increasing sensual pleasure at the expense of the more natural human input, but we know that technological aids can enhance our relationships with others and with ourselves. In this chapter we shall guide you in the use of some of these household items to increase your general health, relaxation, and sensual awareness. In Chapters 8 and 9 we will specifically tell you how to use these devices in working upon the sexual problems or dysfunctions you may have.

What kinds of modern technological magic are we talking about? Nothing with fibre optics or microchips, nothing requiring an engineering degree. We are merely referring to friendly, pleasurable things like hot tubs, whirlpools, vibrators, massagers, even bathtubs! The idea behind the use of these devices, and others under your control, is primarily to teach your body how to experience more and more sensual pleasure in an increasingly relaxed mood and environment. Notice that we say sensual and not sexual. The distinction we are making here in this chapter suggests an enhancement of bodily pleasure but not specifically leading toward orgasms. Even though many of these same devices may be used to bring you to orgasm, focus your thinking and practice for now on sensual pleasure as an end in itself—and not just as a means to orgasmic pleasure. And don't worry, in Chapter 8, we will concentrate more specifically on the orgasmic function.

We are taking the sensual road to sexual fulfillment because of a belief that is shared by many people. The theory goes that people who practice sensual pleasuring often and over many years have a much easier time reaching climax. They even experience a shorter waiting time for sexual response and climax because their bodies and minds are so used to the experience. Subtle tricks are used to maximize stimulation, almost unconsciously because these people know their own bodily responses so well. In a sense, they are maestros of their pleasure organs, rather than inhibited amateurs. As we discussed in Chapter 3, it has been suggested that one of the reasons why males seem less likely to have orgasm problems is that they stimulate themselves more often at a young age than do females. The boys have it much easier. While they are practicing their masturbation, they have less guilt about it because they often brag about it with other boys. Unlike the girls, there is male group support for self-pleasuring. Also, because the male genitalia are external, a young man is used to touching himself when he urinates or bathes and he tends to know what this instrument of pleasure looks like in all stages of arousal. Girls are far less likely to have equal familiarity with their genitalia. Nonetheless, not all men have an easy time of self-pleasuring, so we write this to help both men and women fulfill themselves physically, to achieve what their bodies are capable of feeling sensually.

Another objective of this lesson in self-pleasure is to help men and women reduce the anxiety of sexual performance with others. They often measure their performance by the feedback their partner gives them and they are usually their own toughest critics. To many of these persons, low self-pleasure can thus reinforce the fear that they do not have any "sexual feelings" at all. It is sad to see many people suffer from this when in almost all cases, it can easily be treated and cured. Sometimes we must remind ourselves that we are all sensual beings and we can all train our bodies to better appreciate our sensual feelings. Let us begin with the simplest device of all.

Mirrors

One useful suggestion that we have made is to use a mirror. If you don't already own one, you should buy a hand-held mirror, about 6 to 9 inches across. (If it has an enlarging mirror on the other side, all the better.) With this mirror you can more closely examine your sexual parts and become more familiar with those parts of your anatomy that give you erotic pleasure. Learn to make this association of imagery and sensation, which can be very helpful for later use of fantasy as a means of enhancing arousal and response. So, lie back comfortably, propped up by pillows, and examine your genitals and other parts of your body with the mirror as you touch them. Become as familiar with the look of your genitals as you are with the back of your hand.

Portable Video Cameras

Many people now own one of these small hand-held video cameras that they use when they go on vacations, take home videos of their children's birthday parties, and so forth. The fact that you don't have to send the tape out to be processed, as with the older movie cameras, and the fact that the video can be erased at any time has encouraged some couples to use them in very imaginative ways. For our purposes, in this chapter, we suggest that you use one in the same way that you might use a mirror. Get to know and appreciate your body as it might be seen from the eyes of your spouse or lover. Discover your best features. Look at your facial and body gestures.

Practice the kind of look that you want to project to your love partner. If you are not satisfied with the way you look or sound when you are turned on, change it. It is within your control. Become the film star, the hero or heroine you imagine yourself to be. There is nothing wrong with a little bit of acting.

Sex is not only to carry out the Biblical injunction to be fruitful and multiply. It is also a joyous experience and you should have fun as well as pleasure. First act more playful, then you'll be more fun in bed. Remember, as social psychologists have long said: "Behavior can modify attitudes and feelings." When you behave in a certain way, you will begin to start feeling that way. If you start behaving sexier when you are alone with yourself, you will start to feel more sexy about yourself.

Learn to become comfortable with your own image and those different poses, gestures, and facial expressions that will help make you appear more seductive and alluring. You may even find that making these very personal videos is a definite turn-on. A little bit of narcissism is good for one's ego! Later on, you might consider using the video camera for an erotic turn-on when you are with your spouse or lover. Try to be an exquisite director of romantic and sensual films for your own very private viewing.

Body Mapping

Now, which part of your body is "erogenous?" That is, the rubbing or stimulation of which parts of your body will provide you with that erotic and arousing sensation that makes you want more and more. It would be foolish to talk about "zones" or areas that are common to everybody outside of the obvious genital areas. Practically every part of the body, even the belly button, may produce erotic sensations when touched—from the stroking of hair to the touching and sucking of toes. It all depends upon who is doing it, how, when, and where. It is very important to get to know your own body's likes and be able to communicate them. Therefore, you should touch and stimulate yourself, within practical limits, in all parts of your body, with bare hands, with oils, massagers, vibrators, etc. Later, your partner should help touch and stimulate you in these erogenous areas you have discovered and in a few more places you couldn't successfully reach.

It is important to realize that no two men or women are identical in the erotic intensity of each part of the body. This is because eroticism is not merely a matter of nerve endings; it is also a matter of perception. We know, for example, that for the woman, the nerve endings that produce erotic sensations are only in the outer third of the vaginal entrance. But this is not as important as how the woman *perceives* sensation in the remaining two thirds if they too are stimulated. If she is equally or more responsive to the deeper parts of the vagina, then she should relax and enjoy receiving stimuli there. If a man gets turned on when his wife rubs her breasts across his bald head—wonderful, for him. It doesn't matter if you believe you are the only one in the world who enjoys a certain kind of stimulation. It's your body. Only you know the sensations you feel, so learn as much as you can about that wonderful body of yours.

Think of your entire body as a mapmaker thinks of the planet Earth. You, and later your partner, will begin to map out the different types and degrees of erotic sensations you get from exploring every inch of your body. And just as mapmakers have kept refining maps over the years, after more exploration, you should keep on exploring your own body, at times with the help of others, to know every inch of the "erotic" road! You might want to chart and rate the intensity of the erotic sensations for each part of your body: "the inner thigh rates a 5, the back of the neck a 4, the nipples a 10," and so on. Later, when you are working to bring yourself to orgasm through self-stimulation or when teaching your partner how to bring you to greater orgasms, start with lower levels of stimulation and proceed upward until all the "10" areas are being stimulated.

Vibrators and Massagers

How can you best "map out" your body? We think that the best way is to use a vibrator. We are not talking about using a vibrator to excite the clitoris and bring on an orgasm (see Chapter 8), but rather, for both men and women, using the vibrator to become more aware of how your skin sensitivity varies in each part of the body. The use of a vibrator, in this case, merely multiplies the effect of touching lightly in each area. For instance, if you were to touch the area just below your armpit with your fingers and gently rub in a circular motion, you will probably experience a very pleasant, somewhat erotic sensation. If you try the same thing with a vibrator, you will notice how much more you will feel the sensation. And, if a sexy partner were to use the vibrator on you in the same spot, you will probably experience the sensation even more pleasurably.

Which vibrator should you use out of all the types on the market? We believe that for this "exploratory" phase, the most useful and versatile type is, luckily, the easiest one to buy. They are usually just called "massagers," and you can find them in most outlets and in several mail-order catalogs available nationwide. They look a little like the portable electric mixers you hold in your hand when you beat a cake batter. Instead of the metal mixing attachments, however, there are small attachments or adapters good for massaging the scalp, face, or small areas of the body. Don't get the one that also provides deep heat, because that often becomes a distraction if you are using it to discover the most sensitive parts of your body. But do make sure there is an attachment that is about 1–½ inches in diameter with a convex surface for broader areas of skin, or an attachment that is about ¾ inch long and shaped like a skinny egg for more precise identification of tiny places on the body that arouse you. With luck, you can find a vibrator that has both attachments.

There are other kinds of vibrators or massagers available, but for exploration of your body we believe the "pistol grip" or "portable mixer" type is the most useful. Two other types of massagers that are readily available in department stores and through the major mail-order catalogs are the "Swedish"-type hand massagers and the "wand" type. The wand has a cylindrical handle about 12 inches long, with a vibrating knob on the end that looks like a door knob or a slightly flattened tennis ball. It can be used in a number of ways for erotic arousal, but for this chapter we only want to point out that it is probably the best type for giving yourself (or others) a relaxing massage and increasing your body's sensual awareness. The wand is designed to massage parts of your back as well. There are also attachments that you can buy for it that can enhance its use for sexual excitation. These massagers are used all over the world, so it is not surprising that major international companies like Panasonic and Hitachi make them. Oster makes a rechargeable model as does Wahl.

The "Swedish"-type (sometimes called the back-of-the-hand massager) has been around the longest and has been used by professional masseurs for many years. Sometimes barbers use this type to relax the face and neck muscles of a customer after a haircut and shave. It is not too easy to use on yourself, except on the front of the body. Because of its weight and because it is strapped on over the hand, it is too awkward to use anywhere on one's back. It is fine to use on another person's back. Its greatest value lies in the fact that the vibrations of the motor are transferred to your fingertips. The vibrating effect of your fingers magnifies the sensitivity that the massaged skin feels, and most people prefer to be massaged by human fingertips rather than something artificial. We think you should try all the types of massagers and see which you like best. You may find that each device has its good and bad points for different parts of the body.

There is a new type of vibrator that has recently been developed. It is called the Eroscillator. It is more highly specialized, and, we believe, is the best for stimulation of the labia and clitoris. The Eroscillator is small, only 7 inches in length, and shaped like an electric toothbrush with an oscillating head and a variable speed motor. While it cannot be used for wider massaging and muscle relaxation, it is so effective at narrowly focused stimulation of sensitive parts of the body that you might want to experiment with it. You may certainly want one when you begin the exercises to stimulate the clitoris (described later in Chapter 8).

There is one other common type of vibrator, but most women we have talked to did not get much out of it. This is the type that you might see in a sleazy porno store window, the ones shaped like an erect penis. They seem to be more the product of male fantasy than designed for effective use by women. While they may turn on some people, they are not generally considered to be as effective as any of the models described above.

Before we go on, please note a word of caution! If you buy a massager from a reputable store or mail-order service, there will probably be a paragraph in the instruction booklet that will warn you not to use the vibrator or massager on areas of the body that are swollen. You are also not to use it on the calf of your leg, if you have any pain there. These are wise precautions to maintain because sometimes these pains or unknown swellings may conceal a blood clot that could break loose and harm you. If you have any questions about massaging any pains or swellings do ask your physician. You don't necessarily have to tell the doctor that you are going to massage your clitoris or surrounding area (unless that is where the pain or swelling is). So many people use massagers to relax their muscles after a hard day's work that there is no oddity these days about people wanting to use one.

Some of the devices we have discussed are good for mapping out the most sensitive areas of your body—particularly the portable mixer look-alike—while others are best used to increase your appreciation for your body's sensitivity to touch and pleasure. This will help get you accustomed to allowing and welcoming more bodily pleasure—a total body pleasure that can be erotic and not merely genital.

More than the finest mechanical devices on the market, you need the skills to get your body to relax. Relaxation, mentally and physically, reduces pleasure-destroying stress, as we talked about in the last chapter. We are here suggesting massage, by yourself or better yet with the help of a partner, as a very convenient and fun way of relaxing. Make it a regular part of your routine, become increasingly used to the relaxed state and you will gradually learn to combine massage with meditation or the "relaxation response." This will help prepare your mind and body for increased enjoyment of the sexual act.

O.K., you bought one or more of these massagers and want to know how best to use them. As we said in the previous chapter, you need to set aside a time for privacy when you are not going to be interrupted. Make the room as comfortable and as warm as you can. Splash on a little scented oil or massaging oil, or whatever you might use to pamper yourself. Why not? You deserve it—this is your body you want to give more pleasure to. Take about 15–20 minutes a few times a week for these sessions. They will get better as you make them routine.

But make sure that negative thinking and stress factors don't interfere with your pleasure. Don't think that these exercises are only for people who have problems. All men and women can benefit from these exercises, even if they may have the most fantastic orgasms in the world. Everyone's appreciation of his or her sexuality is enhanced by increased sensitivity to the total body.

When these exercises help you become more sensitive and more relaxed, you will be better able to communicate this to your partner and your sexual relationship will benefit. If you do have any problems with sexual functioning, like the ones mentioned at the beginning of this book, these exercises will help you catch up to where you want to be by preparing you for the sexually oriented exercises to be explained later. So, what we are suggesting here is not therapy as such; it is enhanced appreciation for your body, and something you will want to do for the rest of your life and to encourage others to do for themselves. It is for the pleasure and relaxation of your body, but not as foreplay to an orgasm.

Later on, you may want to use similar techniques of sensual massage for accelerating and enhancing an orgasm, but please don't get confused now. We want you to learn to please and pleasure your body without sexual climax always being the implicit goal. Later, when you apply what you learned about yourself toward specifically sexual and orgasmic goals, you will have to educate your partner about your body, your likes and dislikes. Ignore the old myth that men have this instinctive ability to please the women they really love. This is pure nonsense. Each woman is different and each woman's body must be learned by a man who begins a sexual relationship. Without instructions from the woman, it is fumble and grope, hit and miss, until maybe, *maybe*, he stumbles on her likes and dislikes.

And the same is true for each woman. Your knowledge of what your male partner likes and where his body is sensitive depends to a large degree on his learning about his own body. Each partner in a relationship must take responsibility for his or her own pleasure and responsiveness. So, let the education process begin!

Water, the Great Aphrodisiac

There are some other new devices we want you to consider experimenting with, which will also help enhance your sensual appreciation by enabling you to have other ways to relax and stimulate your entire body. The first of these you can buy fairly inexpensively and install in your bathroom—even if you live in an apartment.

Shower Massagers

The shower massager is a replacement for the conventional shower heads that you will find in any shower. You simply unscrew the old head and screw in the massager head. It is that simple. Yet these gadgets are quite different from ordinary shower heads. First, the head usually has an adjustable pulsator. This allows the water to flow over your body in pulses rather than as a steady stream. This action, similar to certain types of massagers, can have a very soothing and sensual effect on the body. Also, you can vary the intensity of a steady stream from a fine needle-like spray to a heavy downpour.

The second advantage of the shower massager is that its head is attached to a portable handle. You may simply unclip the shower head and move the water spray to any part of your body. The warm pulsations can be aimed within an inch or two of, or directly at, your most intimate parts, if you so desire. Try adjusting the spray to a fine sensual mist and directing it at your genitals and other areas of your body. You are sure to learn about new sensations that your body is capable of responding to. (Some people use these gadgets in the shower to reach orgasm by self-stimulation. That is fine, but for now, just use it for total body stimulation and relaxation and to learn more about your body's sensuality. Wait until Chapter 8 before using it for achieving orgasm. We know you can't wait until you reach Chapter 8, but be patient—one step at a time!)

Hot Tubs

One of the oldest ways of relaxing, going all the way back to Greek and Roman days, was to sit in a warm bath. These were not the tiny bathtubs we usually have in houses and apartments, but great big tubs that several people used at the same time. Many people in the military service who were stationed in Japan after World War II remember how popular they were there, where entire families often went in together. They were not bathing to get clean, since they usually took showers before they went in, but just to get into the very warm water and soak, sometimes for hours at a time.

It seems that some bright people in this country felt that this would be a great idea for us and so the boom in hot tubs began in the Sixties. They first sprung up on the West Coast, where the climate is so much warmer, but now they are more common everywhere, indoors and outdoors. They often use the kind of heating systems employed in swimming pools. A typical hot tub may be 6 to 10 feet in diameter with benches placed on the inside so that you may sit with the water level no higher than your shoulders. Since the water is electrically heated, some people use it year round. They love the effect of sitting outside in warm water during the cold winter. It not only is very relaxing but you are pampering your body and increasing your awareness of its sensitivity in this watery environment.

For a great way to help overcome some of your social inhibitions try inviting friends to join you in your hot tub. You can enjoy this sensuous experience together—even in the nude if you like, as they do in other countries—without necessarily having any sexual overtones. Of course, if you want to add this to your repertoire of presexual activities with a lover, that is alright too (but not until you have finished with all the exercises in this book). Think of what you will have to look forward to after a tense day at work! Because an outdoor hot tub might be the perfect place for a romantic meltdown, make sure you have adequate privacy from your neighbors. Even with no romance in mind the hot tub will probably become your destination after many a hard day's work. Hot tubs are especially effective after dark, with soft lights in the background, soft music, and perhaps even some really good chocolates, like truffles. A little wine might be nice too, but please very little because too much alcohol while you are in a hot tub is not wise. But above all: Relax and enjoy!

Whirlpools

There is a wide range of whirlpools. You might get a device inserted into your current bathtub to create jets of circulating air through the water. You might buy a larger bathtub already equipped with these jets. The larger hot-tub-sized whirlpools are usually called "spas"; they can accommodate from 3 to 6 people. These whirlpools are usually installed indoors, where they take the place of the regular bathtub. In addition to all the benefits and uses that we mentioned in this chapter about bathtubs and hot tubs, whirlpools have added advantages. They allow you to place various parts of your body right in front of the jets so that you get a powerful water massage. This could be very erotic depending upon which part of the body is stimulated. These household whirlpools have developed from the kinds that athletes and patients with muscular problems have used for many years in clinics, clubhouses, and hospitals for the rehabilitation of injured or strained muscles. They have many beneficial effects on the body and they certainly do feel good. Why not double the sensuality and therapy of a whirlpool by sharing the experience with a loved one.

Have Vibrator, Will Travel

Someone told us recently about people who have a "pleasure kit" that they take with them whenever they go on a trip or on vacation. In a large camera bag they pack a set of their sensual "toys": two types of vibrators—a pistol-grip type and an Eroscillator, a "Swedish"-type massager—a latex dildo, scented body oil, massaging oil, a candle, incense, a bottle of wine, and some bubble bath. We think this is a great idea. Just use your imagination and fill up your own pleasure kit with whatever turns you and your partner on! And, if appropriate, don't forget to add a pack or two of condoms—in different colors, to match the sheets. A vacation is an ideal setting for trying out some of the gadgets in this chapter or renting that place with the hot tub.

Why do we need so many gadgets and stimulation devices? It is just plain common sense! A message we want to get across to many readers is: *Don't Complain* about how dull your sex life is! So many men and women, talk about—or feel, but are afraid to talk about—the physical side of their marriage having become so boring. But they do so little about it. We are offering steps to take and "prescriptions" for things to get.

Exercises in increasing yours and your partner's sensual awareness can certainly help make things a little better. They are not solutions in themselves, but in the totality of a stable, monogamous relationship, they will certainly help. Meeting the problem with a plan of action has the secondary effect of helping you take control over your life. When you complain and do nothing, you make yourself psychologically weaker and less able to cope. Inertia begets more inertia. It is as if you were saying to yourself: "Nothing will change, so why bother?" We would rather you say to yourself: "There may not be a miracle cure, but I am going to help deal with the problem of sexual boredom within my relationship, on some meaningful level, in some direct manner." You will then be more like the Captain who comes to take charge of the ship in a storm, and problems of physical boredom are as inevitable as bad weather even in the best of marriages. We know it sounds corny to some people but we believe that everyone should adopt as a motto, the famous line describing that wonderful person, Eleanor Roosevelt: "She would rather light a candle than curse the darkness."

CHAPTER 6

Erotic Arousal Through Make-Believe

So far, we have given you the ability to make an educated guess as to whether or not you or your partner may have a sexual dysfunction. Then, we suggested that, before directly working on any sexual problem or consulting a sex therapist, you learn to control the stress and anxiety that may be causing the sexual misfunctioning. And later, in the previous chapter, we discussed how your entire body may be trained to become even more sensitive and appreciative of sensual stimulation.

If you have diligently followed some of our suggestions, you are now ready to focus in from the sensual to the more specifically sexual. You are now ready for the most important source of sexual arousal—the human brain. That's right! We believe the greatest—and perhaps only—aphrodisiac lies right there between your ears. We know that love and lust and anticipation and tenderness are all very wonderful turn-ons. By all means, they supersede anything else we are talking about in this book. But what should you do when these do not seem to be as effective for turning you on as they once were? We still believe, as most people do, that in the best of all possible worlds—when you love someone—you will feel that deep passion welling up inside, and think about what you are going to do to your spouse or partner: beginning with tenderness and affection and love, and welling up into an overwhelming sexual passion. When this does occur, it is wonderful. There is nothing better!

But even though the brain is not a battery-operated gadget, it still may need some recharging now and then. For many people, particularly after many years of sex with the same person, the old excitement is just not there in the same degree and needs a little assistance. That is what this book is all about, and particularly this chapter. We want to teach you how to use your mind to stimulate the sexual urges *before* there is any physical contact. In other words, you should learn how to put yourself in a sexually receptive mood at will, to make yourself a more erotically oriented person by only using your mind. What do we mean by this?

There is an old joke that we often hear and retell in one

form or another. It goes like this: A young woman during the Czarist period in Russia tells her mother that she is frightened at the thought of her wedding night just a few days away. She doesn't know what to do or what to say to her new husband when they get married. She doesn't know what to do sexually or even how to feel. Her mother tries to reassure her and says, "Don't worry my daughter. Everything will be fine. When your husband comes to you and it is time for him to climb into bed with you, just lie back and think of Mother Russia and the Czarina."

This may not be very funny for some of you, but think of the significance of this old story. If something is unpleasant, we are to use our minds to tune out the experience by concentrating on something that is totally unrelated. This suggests, too, that the opposite is also true. You can use your mind to get more *deeply* involved in a sexual experience, if you so choose. It is up to you which way to go!

You must learn, through practice and more practice, to use your brain to reverse any negative thinking about sex that you may have been brought up with. This is a skill, like any other skill, and it can be learned. It will then become available to you when you want to create your own erotic mental setting around the physical act that takes place. By using some of the techniques we describe in this chapter, you can make your mind work for you. These exercises will help you take charge and be in control over your own newly heightened sensual and sexual sensitivities and skills. You should bring with you all the techniques and procedures of our previous chapters, but remember that your brain is the most important part of your sexual arousal.

Your mind can become like a VCR (video cassette recorder) where you have stored a series of thoughts, fantasies, images, settings, and so forth, which you will play on the screen of your consciousness when you want to. For example, let's say that you saw a movie a few days ago and there was a scene that was especially erotic and arousing to you. You should record or store that scene in your brain and play it back frequently during the next few weeks. It may be used to help you get aroused, or even to help you desire sex when you don't feel especially interested.

If you play back this scene a few times in your mind when you are resting by yourself or taking a break from work, you will be less likely to forget it. You then have an effective "cassette" or memory to pull out when you would like to have sex but do not have as strong an urge as you would like. Playing this "cassette" in your mind should trigger an arousal response that might not otherwise spontaneously appear. This technique helps you be more "horny" when you want to feel that way. By carrying around a figurative shelf full of such "cassettes" in your mind, you will very likely become a more "sexy" person to yourself and *that* is necessary when you want to be sexy for someone else. In other words, you are as sexy as you feel.

What we are suggesting here is that you should not wait for someone else to "turn you on." You should turn yourself on—regularly and frequently—and you may discover that it becomes easier and easier to become spontaneously aroused.

Storing these visually erotic images in your mind is one of the arousal "tricks" that are not dependent on physical contact from someone else or your self-pleasuring. Later (again in that famous Chapter 8) you may use these "mental" motivators as a prologue to physical sexual stimulation. For now let's develop the mental skills in a wide variety of ways for future use. After a while, when you get good at this mental stimulation, you may want to combine these erotic images with the physical stimulation mentioned in the previous chapter. That will be an important step for you: to learn to make an automatic and simultaneous connection between physical and mental arousal.

Let us examine some of the common means of erotic arousal that don't require physical touching. These are visual cues, that is photos and movies, and also the reading of erotic poetry and novels. We are not necessarily endorsing the use of these, since we know that many people have strong feelings about what they may call pornography. We strongly condemn violent, exploitative, and sexist pornography but there is more romantic, less offensive erotica that can help many people. There is much erotica—movies, photos, art work, and novels—which is sensitive and beautiful, and does not contain those negative aspects of the "cheap" pornography. Most librarians know the difference between classic erotica and low-grade pornography, and can steer you to literature or art books of the former type. Also, many of the larger video stores now stock "couples oriented" erotic movies as opposed to the male-oriented X-rated movies. Some of these adult films recommended for couples are even presented from a feminist perspective with an eye to love and romance rather than repetitious male-oriented sex scenes.

Literature and Art

We know today that it is not only men but also women who get aroused by sexually explicit material. This goes beyond movies to include photos and books. The classic *Lady Chatterly's Lover* may be one of the best known novels that has resulted in people getting turned on. Why? Because it is not merely graphic in sexual descriptions, but it is a deeply engaging and fascinating romantic story. It permits you to exercise your imagination and fantasy in identifying with either the male or female protagonist in the story. There are many other sexually explicit romantic novels available in almost every supermarket and discount store today. The woman on the commuter train reading one of these romantic novels may be erotically charging her mental batteries and, consciously or not, helping the sexual dimension of her marriage. Of course, these paperbacks are not in the league of a *Lady Chatterly's Lover*, but if it turns you on—go for it!

We are not trying to suggest that women are more likely to need these formula romance stories to accompany their erotic arousal. The popularity of this genre among women is probably still a carry-over from the puritanical and Victorian attitudes of the past, which denied the legitimacy of inherent female sexual desires. But, if the causes of female sexual repression are rooted in the past, it is interesting to note how many of these novels involve taking us back to a different time period and to faraway places. The exoticism permits us to exercise our fantasies even more, as we safely identify with something far removed from our everyday life. The further these romantic settings are from reality, the less likely they are to trigger a stress-associated thought that would inhibit the erotic response. Remember that stress is to sex what water is to fire. When reading this erotic literature, let your mind freely identify with the character who is having the erotic experience. It is O.K. to get aroused by these books or movies. Then put your lover opposite you in the role of the partner in these erotic acts and self-consciously allow yourself to get turned on. The more you do this, the more you will associate your partner with the erotic and arousing experience. You are teaching your mind and body to become more erotic, and it is amazing how quickly the mind-body learns pleasurable things.

In many ways, even the poorer imitations of great cinematography and great literature, which some people would say have "no redeeming social value," can be of limited educational value to many people developing their sexual interests and awareness. One isn't born a fully developed sexual being, with likes and dislikes and skills and fantasies—one is only born with a partially developed sexual apparatus and a *potential* for sexual magnificence. A person's sexual capability must be nurtured and trained, harnessed and exercised, before we can begin to maximize the pleasures of our love-related sexual experiences. In this sense, because it probably did not happen to us as children or even as teenagers, we need ongoing training as adults to become more sexually interested and more sexually skilled. Sometimes, a grade B novel or a poor adult movie allows us to move ahead to finer things and more enriching sexual food for the mind.

While reading a very good book recently by Edward Brecher, *Love, Sex and Aging,* we were struck with a rather sad situation on the part of some older persons. Many of them had essentially turned off their sexual desires for their spouses as they got older. There was no physical reason for this, but they *believed* that sexual desire wanes after the children are grown. They said, "I don't need it. I can live without it."

In effect, their own minds turned off that very vital part of their marriages, the pleasure of their own eroticism. Some of them who did not have sex for the five to twenty years before their spouses died, suddenly discovered when they met someone new that they were sexually alive and well. Eroticism doesn't run out when the social security rolls in!

Their sexual interest and desires hadn't disappeared while their longtime spouses were alive; it just became buried under the misconception that he or she has no more sexual urges. We are not suggesting that married people who feel that they have lost their sexual urges go out and find someone else to rekindle the old spark. But such people, and that may well include *you,* must produce and direct the mental set and script to make your sex life vibrant, to take active control in developing new sexual awareness and interest within the relationship. While some people may want to "label" this problem as "sexual desire dysfunction," it may not be as serious as it seems. Before you decide to go to a therapist, try to help yourself through relaxation, stress reduction, pleasure-inducing "gadgets," and *your own mind*—and with a few more suggestions from us that we will tell you about. Don't complain—take charge! There is nothing wrong or shameful about going to a sex therapist, but it shouldn't be your first course of action. If what we are saying and suggesting here doesn't work for you, then you might need the expertise of a therapist to find out what may be blocking you from achieving your sexual goals. Remember, there is nothing magical about what a sex therapist does. He or she has no high-tech machines to wire you up to or miracle drugs to prescribe as an aphrodisiac. Much of a good therapist's help is plain common sense, the same sort of advice we are giving you here.

Adult Movies

As we said earlier in this chapter, we recognize that many of the available "adult" movies and videos are little more than trash. But in the last five years or so there has been a greater shift on the part of some adult movie producers toward romantic love stories that are also sexually explicit. These high-quality, well-written and -acted films might only have one or two of these sexually explicit scenes. It seems that these producers have come to realize that if they want to attract a female audience or to make movies that couples can feel comfortable watching together, they have to do two things: 1) Be more sensitive to the woman's perspective and not merely cater to male fantasies, and 2) They have to produce a more artistic production of an X-rated film, one with an interesting story line, fine cinematography, and good acting. Some of these "adult" movie producers and directors have succeeded but, unfortunately, these movies usually get lost amidst the trashy stuff. The best way to find out about them is to ask the video store owners. Many of them know which ones are of high quality and not offensive to women and couples.

While many of these "adult" movies are exclusively heterosexual in orientation, some of them also show two women or two men making love. If we can judge by the number of films that are rented that show women making love to each other in a primarily heterosexually oriented movie, men seem to get turned on by watching women making love to each other. On the other hand, there are few heterosexual movies available in video stores that show men engaged in sex with each other. Only rarely do women report being turned on by watching men engaged in homosexual acts in these adult videos.

Another interesting observation made by sex researchers is that both men and women, who have no inclination for any sexual contact with people of their own sex, may get turned on by watching two people of their own sex, engage in a homosexual act on the screen. For them, as long as this turn-on is limited to the screen, it is a safe, "exciting" turn-on that they will not try themselves. This also may apply to a variety of taboo acts often appearing in adult videos. From our point of view, as long as watching these exotic, different, and "forbidden" acts remains as visual images only (and there is a wide range of heterosexual acts that are equally taboo), these films could be used to enhance one's sexual excitement.

It seems reasonable that adults may watch these movies in the privacy of their own homes, and the law protects our right to do so. Now, if there are some scenes or movies that are distasteful, don't watch them. If a particular movie is not arousing, push fast forward and try another video some other time.

Remember, if you do find a scene especially erotic, go back and look at the scene over and over again until you have a vivid picture etched into your brain. By doing this, especially if you do this by yourself, you are educating your mind into a more sexual orientation and that should help you in your physical arousal. Later on, when you are with your partner, you may recall a particular scene for foreplay arousal. But for now just watch these movies and scenes by yourself in order to make your mind more erotically receptive through vicarious imagery.

When you watch these erotic movies by yourself, to enhance your erotic capabilities, create a romantic and receptive mood—for *you*—before you turn on the VCR. Approach these viewing sessions as if you were beginning a meditation session: Use time periods when you know you won't be disturbed, dim the lights, take the phone off the hook, and sit or lie down in a comfortable spot. Make sure you don't have to interfere with the viewing by doing the laundry, or worrying that you really should be grocery shopping or something else. Make sure you don't have the noise of a washing machine or dishwasher to distract you. You will want to create a romantic mood, even though you are alone for these sessions. You might light some incense, if that is what you like, or have some wine, light a few candles, or whatever makes you feel romantic. Because you want to create a mood that is conducive for your identification with the male or female lead in a romantic sex movie, provide yourself with the setting to get into the movie as much as possible. You want to become so receptive to the action that you bond with the feelings and actions of the actor or actress during the erotic acts shown on the screen. Your viewing cannot be completely passive or purely intellectual if it is to have the effect upon you that you need. You cannot view it as if you were viewing a sunset because that kind of activity is oriented to make you tranquil and appreciative—not erotically aroused. But now you want to be an active participant in the action of the movie, even if it is only in your mind. You cannot be stuffing popcorn into your mouth while sitting on a metal folding chair and wonder why that great sex scene isn't doing anything for you. You have to *actively* view the scenes by engaging your mind and relating your body sensations to what is happening in the movie. When a scene is especially arousing, we want you to *imagine* that your spouse or partner is the other person in the movie involved in the sexual acts. When such a scene appears and you are really turned on by it, *turn off* the video and relive the scene *in your mind*. Picture you and your lover in this role and act it out over and over again in your *fantasy*. Soon enough, you will be bringing this cinematic energy into your flesh-and-blood love life.

Imagery and Fantasy

Which came first: the chicken or the egg? Who cares, as long as you know how to cook! So, what does this age-old riddle have to do with sexual interest and erotic arousal? Well, does your interest in sex cause you to become more easily aroused, or, are you more interested in sex because you are so frequently and strongly aroused naturally? Actually, it works both ways. By training yourself to become more interested in sex, you will become more easily aroused, and as you become more frequently aroused you will have a greater interest in sex.

If you think back, you will probably remember something

from the past that really aroused you sexually. Back then, something you had seen, perhaps accidentally, or some situation you were in caused you to become sexually aroused. Put yourself back in your old shoes. Now, think of the same incident with your eyes closed and relive that incident step by step. (Again, do this when you are alone and in quiet, non-disturbing surroundings.) Allow yourself to once again feel the same stirrings and excitement that you felt then. Do this several times in your mind and practice varying it from time to time. Allow the action to go a bit further than it had in reality. Allow yourself to respond in a more uninhibited manner than you might have then. Do things and have things done to you that you would never dream of doing in reality.

Now, imagine yourself watching other people you know in erotic acts or having someone special secretly watching you engaged in uninhibited sex. (Perhaps that person you had a crush on but couldn't meet can help you now, in your mind.) Experiment with different kinds of images and begin to use these images as stage settings in your own mind. You are the producer, director and casting agent. Populate the stage with whomever you choose and have them and you, the star, do anything you have secretly thought would be a great turn-on but did not dare to do in reality. You are now fantasizing, using your mind to interest and arouse your body in an erotic direction. Always bear in mind that these are learning experiences for you, to explore safely within your own mind. Open yourself to the widest possible range of images that may turn you on, so that you can use them to sharpen your sexual interests and desires and make erotic responses that much easier to have when you are with someone.

You started out this exercise by remembering a sexually arousing experience from the past, your first and deepest impression perhaps. We now want you to create altogether new scenarios with which to *begin, maintain and enhance* your erotic arousal. And this is wonderful! You are now taking control of arousing yourself (and not even by touching yourself in any auto-erotic manner). You will soon build up a repertoire of fantasies that you can use whenever you need one. They tend to stay in your mind for easy reference, yet no one need know about them. They are your mental toys—the only true aphrodisiacs we know of. In these fantasies, you can repeat a favored plot but substitute any person you want. You can thus change the subtleties of the same mental-erotic experience.

In the fantasy world you can put in persons who are absolutely forbidden or unavailable to you. Some people have said that fantasy seems to work best for erotic arousal when the object of your fantasy is someone you know but who is forbidden to you. There are many people who fantasize about movie stars or others whom they can probably never even see in person. You might fantasize about your favorite rock star or singer but we think it is probably best if your fantasy person is a real live person. Too much romantic or erotic attention to an idealized movie star or entertainer can easily become boring if there is no contact at all between you. Better you should make someone whom you see in the flesh at least once in a while the object of your fantasy.

Your fantasy person should live somewhere in the realm of possibility, although be very unattainable. But of course, if you so desire, you can fantasize about two lovers at the same time, or three, or an entire football team or cheerleader squad! We have much more mental than physical energy. There are no limits, as long as you realize that fantasies *must* stay in your mind. There are some people who try to act out their fantasies in real life. Sometimes, it works but probably, more often, our inability to control real-life situations may present some serious hazards.

Should you ever tell your lover which fantasy is going on in your head? Probably not. For some people, sharing a fantasy with their spouses or lovers can be good and it may turn them both on. Only you can determine if they would enjoy or resent such mental sex play. So, always use your common sense and, if anything, err on the side of caution when it comes to telling others about your fantasies.

The Sex Break

Now you have all these "mental" arousal skills and a visual "library" of erotic scenes in your head. You even had some practice in calling up these images and relating them to bodily sensations. You now have to practice these wonderful new skills in a more routine manner. Why practice these mental images and fantasies? We think that practice is very important for most people, because, as social psychologists have so often told us, behavior can affect attitude as much as attitude affects behavior. When it comes to problems of lagging sexual interest and desire, we might look at these as attitudes and try to change them as we would any set of attitudes. Thus, if you begin to act as if sex was one of the most natural, non-threatening, and important things in your life, we believe that your attitudes and feelings will change accordingly.

What we are suggesting here is making a ritual or institution—in your personal life—of a *sex break*. What is a sex break? Essentially, it is the same thing as a coffee break at work or at home. To us, if sex isn't at least as important as a cup of coffee, something is very wrong with our cultural values. Besides, caffeine is an unhealthy stimulant drug that can give you heartburn or worse, and the cake or doughnuts you probably have with it only put on unnecessary and unhealthy pounds. So, down with the coffee break and up with the sex break!

Where do you take a sex break? At the cafeteria or doughnut shop? Only in your head, of course. If you are at work, at home, in a train, or plane, after skiing, or whatever—take a five-, ten- or even a fifteen-minute break from what you are doing, if possible, and close your eyes. In a sense, it is like the stress-reduction techniques we discussed in Chapter 4. But, instead of emptying the mind of the distracting "chatter" that tends to stress us a great deal, we concentrate on taking out and playing a visual image or fantasy video from our mental repertoire. During the screening we separate the everyday world from this secret world of pleasure that exists in the private theater of our minds. These short breaks are very relaxing and serve to reinforce to ourselves the importance of sex. The more we reinforce it, the more important it will become to us. Our experience has shown that as we place more importance on sex, even when it is only on the intellectual level, our interest and desires grow on the physical and emotional level. But this is only common sense. When do we ever develop much of an interest in something we place very little importance?

One of the by-products of these "sex breaks" is that you will quickly learn to integrate the fantasies and images with the social situations in the real world around you. You will sometimes incorporate the images of a co-worker into your fantasy when you are at work, a neighbor or friend when at home, your spouse or lover while he or she is in the shower, and so forth. These sex breaks are safe as long as you realize that they are to be kept within your psyche and to help you grow in sexual desire and interest. They are not to be a prelude for unwise action in the real world, such as serious flirting with the object of your fantasy desire.

Erotic Dream Programming

One of the best times to use imagery and fantasy is when you are trying to fall sleep. This is the "twilight zone" between waking consciousness and sleep. At these moments, take a few minutes to fantasize. Why use the old method of counting sheep? Fantasy before sleep is more fun and we believe that it works better. It's really a very simple idea, and it is called EDP (erotic dream programming).

When we first heard someone talking about EDP we couldn't figure out what "electronic data processing" had to do with sex. It was later apparent that it was not a computer job title but had something to do with sex and dreams. How do dreams enter the picture? That's the bonus part. If the fantasizing is done correctly, you will find that more and more often you will have dreams related to the fantasy. How do you program your own dreams? After you go to bed, when you are alone and have not yet fallen asleep (if you are with a spouse or partner, then wait until he or she falls asleep), role play a little erotic story in your mind based on some real incident you know of or one you would like to happen. Make it rather brief and uncomplicated. Keep repeating this story over and over in your mind until you fall asleep.

People tell us that they have noticed four beneficial results:

- First, it helps you fantasize more easily when you want to at some other time—especially when you will be with someone during a sex act.
- Second, it helps build the repertoire of fantasies you have stored in your mind for use at later times when you need them.
- Third, these fantasies at bedtime help you fall asleep. They are much better than counting sheep, drinking an alcoholic beverage, or taking a tranquillizer.
- Fourth, if you fall asleep during the fantasy, it is possible that your dreams will be an extension of the fantasy. (This appeals to many people we have talked with who would like to have some control over their dreams.)

Going to bed with your fantasy can help you become a more relaxed person because the process of erotic dream programming is similar to other stress-reduction techniques.

A repeated fantasy works like meditation since role-playing this erotic scenario over and over in your mind will relax the chatter in your head. It pushes out all those anxiety-provoking thoughts about what you should or should not have done during the day. The more familiar your fantasy becomes, the more this technique has the effect of repeating a mantra during the meditation process. But instead of a word, you are using an erotic image or action that you repeat over and over.

Because erotic dream programming is so useful in reducing stress, many people use it when they awaken at three or four o'clock in the morning and can't fall back to sleep. At these times, why worry about falling asleep again, or the fact that you have to get up in a couple of hours, or about all the things you have to do after you wake up? Instead, make this time productive for you by reducing stress and increasing your erotic fantasy skills by engaging in EDP. Call up that favored fantasy scenario and play back an erotic scene over and over again until you fall back to sleep.

Your erotic "mantra" will help you get to sleep, or back to sleep, and it will get rid of the stressful uncontrolled "chatter" in your mind. The more you practice using erotic imagery in this manner, the more likely it will be carried over into the sleep state. As your skill at doing this increases, you will be more likely to have an erotic dream that is related to or may even be a continuation of your fantasy. So, one might say that *erotic dream programming* is not only fun but that it may be good for you both mentally *and* physically. All this, without costing you a penny and while you are lying in bed! Not bad, but there is more.

Erotic dream programming also offers you an opportunity

to explore and expand your erotic interests by experimenting in a very safe manner—inside your own head and in the privacy of your thoughts. EDP can therefore help you develop new interests in the ways and conditions in which you might like to have sex. If you fantasized about an erotic encounter on a beach, rooftop, or in a row boat, perhaps you could maneuver your loved one to such a setting. Even if you cannot fulfill the sometimes impossible aspects of your fantasy, at the very least you are helping to train your mind to think in a more erotic fashion. You are building your interest in sex and recognizing the joys and the healthy practical uses of eroticism. You see, EDP is even educational!

Morning Fantasy

The alarm goes off in your bedroom at 6:45 AM. You reach out to turn it off and then get out of bed to begin another day of work. So wake up, shake the sleep out of your eyes, start doing those calisthenics, and get moving. Sounds familiar? But now we come along and say: *Hold it!* You certainly have responsibilities to your career and family but what about yourself?

If you were one of the few people who were completely satisfied with his or her level of libido and sexual activities, we assume you wouldn't be reading this far. But now that you are, we would like you to spend a very valuable part of the day to help you along in this training process so that you will feel more erotically motivated. And this valuable time is precisely the period just after you wake from a sound sleep. When you are not yet fully awake you are in the morning "twilight zone."

Some people feel that this time is even more important than when you go to sleep at night because a morning fantasy can help set the tone for the rest of the day for you. Even if it's brief, you'll have many opportunities for reinforcement if you take the "sex breaks" we suggested earlier in the chapter.

What exactly should you do in the morning? Essentially the same thing you did the night before, when you did the erotic dream programming with fantasies. Only this time, as you lie in bed, drowsy and comfortable, take a few minutes to create a fantasy involving someone you are likely to see or speak to during the day. That adds a little spice to your forbidden fantasy, and a little more erotic excitement. After all, who knows what may happen during the day? (No, don't plan on acting out on it during the day; fantasy works best only when you leave it at that.)

At this stage, do not touch yourself auto-erotically during the fantasy. As in all exercises during this chapter, you are only trying to exercise, excite, and teach the mind to think of yourself in a more sexy manner. You will have plenty of opportunity for bringing it all together in Chapters 8 and 9. In the meantime, create some interesting and exciting fantasies for yourself for tomorrow morning and many mornings after. Relax and enjoy them before you face the real world. These morning fantasies will be good for your erotic life and help reduce the stress that you, like most people, face every day. Try it, you'll like it!

CHAPTER 7

The Working Woman and Changing Sex Roles

Why such a sociological bent to a chapter heading in a book that is trying to help you enhance your sex life and overcome any sexual dysfunctions? Because some people have problems, including sexual problems, that are shaped and even caused by events in the society around them, events over which they have no real control. In this instance we are referring to changes in the traditional roles of men and women that have occurred in our own adult lifetime. These changes have taken place so rapidly that not all of us have been able to adjust to them. Some of us are bewildered about women who seem to act more in a way typical of what we used to consider men's behavior to be, or men who appear to take on more feminine traits rather than the stereotyped "macho" ones. Consequently, it seems that we often see people who say that they have "sexual problems," but after talking with them it becomes clear that they really have problems in male/female role relationships. They have a role stereotype problem rather than a sexual dysfunction.

These specific problems arise when much of what men and women know about sex and its interpersonal context was learned before the early 1960's. That is, people who had been raised as boys and girls before the turbulent times of the late 1960's and early 1970's, when all these changes in the relationships between men and women developed had to adjust to a different social world and new definitions in the way men and women should behave, after the so-called "sexual revolution" and the women's movement.

In many other cultures today and in America of twenty-five years ago, the woman was *supposed* to have a more passive role while the man was *supposed* to be the aggressor, the initiator of sexual activity. In addition, the husband was *supposed* to be the breadwinner, making his way in the business or professional world, while the traditional wife was at home taking care of the house and children. Strong elements of sexism were present in male-female relations at that time as the woman's passive role meant subordination to the male in most circumstances in life, including sexuality and remunerative work. But today, this is not the reality for most couples. Women usually have to, and want to, work at a profession outside the home, and sexism, which assigns the passive role to the woman, is on its way out.

Younger women don't seem to have the same kinds of problems as their mothers. But women forty and over may still have to learn to give themselves *permission* to initiate sex, and their husbands have to learn to accept their wives as possible initiators of sex without feeling that their masculinity is being threatened. We know that most men like it when a woman initiates sex, but what if a man was raised to believe that a "normal" woman is only sexually interested or sexually excited when a man (her husband, of course) touches her genitals in order to arouse her? He might get very confused or even suspicious of his wife's activities when he is not around. While this is not a problem of sexual dysfunction, as such, it becomes a problem more related to *sexual literacy*. We must now teach him that his old attitudes and knowledge about female sexuality are not only erroneous, but can be very harmful to the sexual aspects as well as the trust component of his marital relationship.

What has compounded this problem is that changes in the traditional role relationships between husband and wife have been forced upon even the very traditional marriages. This is due to the fact that many women have to work in today's economy. The working wife and mother is no longer the exception but is now the norm. This new freedom for women to work beyond the household, however, can present a conflict that is often unrecognized in many marriages. This shift in the work force in our society brought with it a change in many women's personalities. Moving into the labor force to take jobs and develop careers outside the home, women soon learn how important it is to become more assertive and aggressive than they had to be as wives, mothers and homemakers. Thus, these changes in assertiveness affect the self-image of the wife who now sees herself as more capable of being economically independent and a self-determinate decision maker. Almost always, while undergoing these changes in herself, a wife will change the way she relates to others. In particular, this may cause strain in her relationship to her husband who must accept these lifestyle and personality changes, often without understanding them.

For many women, striving and sometimes reaching their goals of becoming more economically independent, working at an interesting full-time job outside the home where she meets new people, having as many job responsibilities as her husband does, does not bring her the sense of complete freedom and equality as much as she might have hoped for. Marian Burros points out in her wonderful new cookbook, *20 Minute Menus,* that for many women, life got harder, not easier:

> As a *New York Times* poll in the fall of 1987 revealed, despite the feminist revolution, women, whether they work outside the home or not, still do most of the cooking and shopping.
>
> Ninety-one percent of all married women shop for food and 90 percent of all married women cook. Eighty-six percent of married women who work outside the home do

the cooking, while 90 percent of the married women who work outside the home do the shopping.

Now, if the traditional husband, with minimal involvement in household chores, knows his wife is working all day, and when she comes home she also takes care of the children, does the food shopping, and cooking, then he should not be surprised if she has a headache or is tired when he makes sexual advances at the end of a typically hectic day. She has every right to be exhausted and to have other concerns on her mind. We are not saying this to justify or condone this kind of all work and no play relationship, but we must be sensitive to the changes that may take place even within the happiest of marriages.

In today's economy not only do most women have to work, but many men have to work harder and longer to increase the family income. As the parody of an old aphorism goes: "Work is the curse of the drinking class." We are also sure that hard work may sometimes interfere with something much more important than drinking: *a desirable sex life.* Some people just allow themselves to become overwhelmed with work and find themselves responding less and less to sexual urges. Too often, even the desires themselves begin to wane.

These lowered sexual drives do not indicate sexual dysfunction problems but are human relations problems that go beyond the bedroom. Without sufficient time and energy, sex may be reduced to an obligatory act—and that is not usually very pleasurable. What can a hardworking couple do? In a few cases they can make some financial sacrifice by cutting down on work or they may cut down some of their bridge, bowling, or even civic activity time for the sake of their sex life and marriage. They might be able to use part of that double income to get some household help for cleaning, shopping, cooking, or childcare. If you have a large enough house or apartment you can often find a college student who will be glad to help out in exchange for free room and board. Taking in needy students was a tradition in Europe for centuries but somehow never really caught on in the United States. Too bad, because in a situation like this everyone benefits: You do a good deed and get help and often you get a new friend in return. Even if more expensive professionals have to be hired and one of your annual vacations has to be downgraded, won't it be worth it for more time and energy to enjoy each other's company every night?

Another consideration that may help is to examine what your expectations are as to how clean and neat you *have* to keep the home. You don't want to create a situation where household drudgery is the price you pay for love, companionship, and marriage. If both partners share equally and you do not demand of yourselves a "white glove inspection" every time there is cleaning to be done, you will have that much more time for the important things in life: your children, your sex life, your creative hobbies, and so forth. It seems to us that women are the victims of the economic pressures of today much more than men because the socially learned female role of responsibility for maintaining the home and nurturing the children was developed at a time in history when women were at home to do the work. But today, to do all this and to work outside the home—to be the Supermom who wants it all—is unrealistic without a lot of help from your partner or significant other. Stop blaming the other person for being tired and not interested in sex. You both work too hard. Don't complain, do something about it!

We know that you probably have heard it a zillion times but it is so important that it bears repeating in this context: *Look at your priorities.* What is most important for you: money, friends, time for your children, time for yourself, sex, intellectual pursuits, creative work, or what? No one can have it all. If you can take a really hard look at yourself and what you really want as opposed to what you were brought up to believe you are *supposed* to want, you might reorganize your life considerably. You might see that you are sacrificing happiness—especially your own—for the sake of a less-than-crucial goal.

For some people we know, this soul-searching has even resulted in a mid-life career change that allows them to more fully be themselves without sacrificing their loved ones. Remember, you will probably have a very long life ahead of you. We just heard some projections that by the beginning of the 21st Century (less than ten years away) the percentage of people over the age of one hundred will be almost six times greater than it is today and the percentage of people over the age of sixty-five will go up from about fifteen to nearly thirty percent of the population. Since most people will be living longer, it's time you straightened out your priorities and planned for the erotically satisfying sex life you can have when your hair is silver. Otherwise, you could be growing older without that special ingredient that creates a sparkle in your eye – good sex.

It is unrealistic to expect that sex will automatically

become exciting again when the last child goes off to college and you have each other alone again. It doesn't work that way. The "empty nest syndrome" can seem even emptier when perfunctory, passionless sex has become the habit. Remember, twenty-five-year habits are very hard to break, so it is best if you make sex an important part of your life *right now*.

What we are suggesting here is that you allow yourselves the best times of the day and week for sex to take place. Make sure that you allow yourselves enough time to permit the sexual desires to be awakened. You may have to go beyond the so-called "foreplay": touching a nipple or clitoris here, stroking a penis there. The old notion that all one needs is sufficient time for foreplay is not always true, especially if there are any sexual difficulties at all or if one or both spouses are tired or under stress. You may have to plan for the best time to allow your psychic energy to build up again, like waiting for the weekend rather than attempt a frustrating "quickie" that can be psychologically damaging if not successful.

For some men and women, a "quickie" is not necessarily bad. That is, if the both of you can achieve sexual gratification during a stolen moment before going out to dinner so that you arrive there like two new lovers sharing a secret—wonderful! While no one is going to suggest that quick sex is ever going to replace the lingering, leisurely lovemaking sessions you enjoy best, if you have the kind of schedule that doesn't permit this as often as you like and the two of you don't have any negative feelings about "quickies," then go for it. And if you plan in advance so neither of you is disappointed, you both don't have to climax in a "quickie" session. You can arrange it so that this time, your husband will lie back and be passive for a few minutes while you pleasure him and—turnabout is fair play—the next time you relax while he does all the work with his fingers or tongue or whatever.

Some women are afraid that because they take many minutes or longer to orgasm, they will never be satisfied during a "quickie." This doesn't have to be so. If you are this woman you can teach yourself to respond more quickly by following many of the suggestions in this book. For one thing while you are contemplating having the "quickie" you can think many erotic thoughts and fantasies while you are doing other things. Then, you can masturbate with your fingers or a vibrator just before your husband touches you and while he is also helping to arouse you. One of the best ways to arouse yourself is for you to do the planning for the "quickie" and surprise your lover by beginning it as soon as you see him without telling him in advance. The anticipation of the surprise is often a strong turn-on itself. The main thing is to have fun during these stolen moments and that they should not be used to only one person's advantage and pleasure.

Another problem we see more of these days also appears related to the newly acquired assertiveness that women learn when they move out into the business world. It seems that many men who were brought up in more traditional times have difficulty coping with their wives' growing assertiveness. We are not referring to the sexual assertiveness discussed at the beginning of this chapter, but a more general assertiveness derived from a woman's day-to-day business or work world. The woman begins to take on the traditional male role, making more decisions and assuming responsibilities that she might have left to the husband at an earlier time.

We find that some men are upset by this, because, without being able to verbalize it, they are confused by their wives doing things that only the husband did before. To put it colloquially, these men worry about "who is wearing the pants in the family." These same men can feel threatened by insignificant things like the woman taking in the car for repairs or negotiating with the bank for a home improvement loan. Even little things like these can affect a man's image of his own masculinity, if he has been traditionally raised. Her "manly" behavior will create some doubts as to whether his wife still thinks of him as the "man" of the house.

We know men who begin to suspect that another man might be behind his wife's emerging independence. These jealous anxieties cannot be good for the marriage or the relationship, and certainly not good for sex. What to do about them? Before consulting a marriage counselor or a sex therapist, take the time to talk to each other about these fears and anxieties. It is amazing how much good some old-fashioned talking with common sense and expressing your feelings openly to your significant other can clear the air. Besides, if you want to reduce or eliminate any sex problems or to improve the quality of your sex life *you have to be able* to express your feelings and talk openly with your partner. Just as we suggested earlier that you rule out stress, physical, and other factors before concluding that you have a problem of sexual dysfunction, we now say that you must also rule out any closed up avenues of communication or strait-jacketed feelings.

CHAPTER 8

What You Can Do for Yourself

This chapter is really divided into two parts: The first part speaks about what women can do for themselves to overcome some of their sexual dysfunction difficulties, while the second half addresses the men. Since we believe that both parts should be read by each sex, we include them in one chapter. This will provide readers of each sex with a better understanding of some of the differences and similarities between the sexual responses of males and females. Even when we discuss a specific method that only applies to one sex, a person of the opposite sex may be able to creatively integrate it within his or her own exercise program.

Women: How to Help Yourselves

Having read this far, you can probably rule out many possible causes for what you may have thought was a sexual dysfunction. You are *now* ready for more advanced erotic training —this time of the genitals—if:

1) You have gotten a grip on the stresses in your life and can now relax.
2) You have practiced your erotic fantasy skill development.
3) You have learned to better appreciate the sensuality of your body.
4) You have trained your mind to think along more erotic lines.
5) You are sure that medications or other drugs are not interfering with your erotic response.

If, after all the suggestions we have made and all the procedures you have followed in the previous chapters, you *still* have no interest in sex with anyone, no erotic dreams and wishes, no pleasurable responses when you touch yourself or someone touches you, or you still have any feelings of revulsion about sex or the genitals, then we suggest that it might be a good time for you to make an appointment with a qualified sex therapist or clinical psychologist to evaluate your problem in more detail. If you want, of course, you can continue to follow the suggestions that apply to you in this later part of the book. We don't want you to think that you are hopeless if you are not the kind of erotic individual you would have liked to be. There is always hope for you to solve your problems no matter how insoluble they appear to be. If we cannot help you ourselves, then some other qualified helping professionals may be able to.

If you think back about what you had been reading in the previous chapters, you will see that we have been presenting a sort of training program. It is a training program for your body and mind, to get you in shape physically and psychologically for maximum sexual enjoyment. These preparatory steps are very much like what skiers do to prepare for the slopes. They must not only do the right warm-ups just before skiing, but they must also keep their muscles toned up and in shape in the summer when they are not skiing. All year long they have to keep the right mental outlook. They read about skiing, talk about it, and even dream about it. True skiers will even fantasize about it. They role-play in their minds the moves they will make as they go from the top of the hill to the bottom. As all skiers know, mental role-playing is a very important part of preparing themselves for the skiing itself. In short, a serious skier's self-image has to be developed and refined over and over again before he or she gets onto the slopes when the new opportunity arises.

And, just as the skier keeps his fanny bag and equipment bags packed, you lovers should keep an erotic bag packed, as we talked about in an earlier chapter. Remember, that love bag is like a ski bag, or a tennis bag, or a camera bag or any other recreational bag. It is for fun and your peace of mind, not for duty or obligation or work!

Now that you have the skills, and that you have the equipment, and the knowledge of all these techniques, and you know how to reduce stress and relax, what comes next? What can you do for yourself to help you overcome the kinds of problems we mentioned in Chapters 2 and 3? Let us begin with one of the common difficulties that we discussed in Chapter 2: women who say that they cannot achieve orgasm.

Difficulty in Reaching Orgasm

We stressed earlier that orgasmic resolution is something a woman feels must take place when there is *sufficient physical stimulation* to bring her to that point. That is, the orgasmic reflex will automatically take over when that point is reached. But the problem is, and it is different for each woman, when and how to reach that point.

There are women who experience difficulty in having an orgasm while using their fingers to stimulate themselves. They continue the effort and begin to feel what they believe is sexual excitement build up but then there is no increase in excitement as they continue to masturbate. This is because increased movement is not the same as increased stimulation. You must interpret for yourself whether any suggestion we make is truly "stimulating" for *you*. The most powerful vibrator could be turned on you without your being turned on by it. Stimulation is the positive erotic effect one feels rather than the source of the possible stimulation.

How much time is needed for erotic stimulation? There is no way that we can suggest a specific number of minutes that would be needed for you to have an orgasm. That varies greatly with each woman and each occasion. What we can say is that you have to plan a daily strategy of varied sources of stimulation and gradually increased amounts of time.

A Plan for Stimulation

Our suggestion is that you begin your strategy with the most common and simplest source of stimulation: your fingers. Plan to start with a few minutes of manual self-stimulation, but only *after* you have created the relaxed and private environment we have spoken about earlier where you are not likely to be intruded upon. While lying down with your knees raised or flat, whichever is more comfortable for you, gently massage the areas around your clitoris for a few seconds to initiate the process. Gently rub below, above, on the right, and on the left of the clitoris. Every once in a while gently massage the clitoris itself. Be fully aware of the sensations you are feeling without trying to consciously think about how you are doing it. Treat this like a meditative experience and just feel the growing excitement. If, after a few minutes, the excitement continues to mount, continue whatever you are doing because you must be doing something right. If at any point you feel that the excitement is waning or has disappeared, then stop. That is your body telling you that it has had enough for the moment.

When you have stopped, reinforce those pleasant sensations by recalling them and what you were doing to achieve that feeling. For the next time when you can exercise the orgasmic reflex, plan to shift a little earlier, in your excitement phase, to another way of stimulating your genitals with your fingers that might help increase the perceived stimulation—perhaps stroking your nipples with the other hand or playing with your anus. See if this raises the excitement level even higher.

Plan to incorporate into your strategy the use of latex dildos to further heighten your excitement and then move on to vibrators and various combinations of techniques. But remember, the goal is increased excitement and does not have to be orgasms in the early stages of your genital stimulation. In other words, your strategy should not specifically revolve around bringing yourself to orgasm, but rather to increase your perceived sensations and pleasure. As excitement grows along with your fantasies, you *allow* the orgasm to come by itself.

Think of it this way. You are creating the *conditions* that permit this wonderful feeling, hidden inside of you, to come to the surface. Look at your explorations and experimentations as a learning model, a sort of biofeedback mechanism, where your brain learns and stores the right movements and fantasies that help you increase the erotic sensations. If you want the old-fashioned non-scientific version of this model, it is: If this doesn't work, then try that, and if that doesn't work, try the other thing and then, to increase the stimulation, try the next thing you think of. No matter how we phrase it, it boils down to the fact that you may have to try a variety of techniques, intensities, and sources of stimulation until you develop a pattern that works for you. You can accomplish this by being sensitive to those techniques that appear to be increasing *your* erotic stimulation and relying less on those techniques that are no longer as effective. Eventually, your repertoire will have exercised the vaginal-clitoral system well enough so that you won't have to work at it to have an orgasm. Remember to concentrate on *pleasuring* yourself, not merely on reaching orgasm. Now, let's get more specific about the different kinds of sources of stimulation.

Your Best Problem-Solving Tool: Masturbation

After creating the necessary atmosphere, slowly stroke yourself all over for a few minutes: your face, thighs, arms, belly, breasts, behind, and wherever else your hands can reach. Then let your fingers slowly circle the area around the clitoris. Move your fingers in and out of the vagina and use the natural lubrication to moisten the outside lips of the vagina as you massage them. Every once and a while, let your fingers gently stroke the clitoris and note your response. If you like the sensation, stroke the clitoris more frequently as you massage around it. Some women don't like to have the clitoris stimulated directly because they perceive it as too intense. But, that is for you to decide. The important thing is not to do anything at this stage unless you are enjoying it and becoming erotically aroused. If you are enjoying the manual stimulation of the vaginal area but are not getting erotically stimulated, don't get disappointed. You should still continue doing it as long as you do receive some pleasure from the stimulation. This is a very valuable learning experience for the stimulation of the orgasmic reflex. Take your time—it will pay off in increased erotic pleasure for the rest of your life.

It is very important that this vaginal and clitoral stimulation be carried out on a daily basis. We know that sometimes it may be impractical to create the quiet, romantic mood we discussed earlier, but every woman should have some private moments during the day. It may be in the morning, before getting out of bed, or in the bathroom while taking a shower or bath, or whatever. The conditions may not be perfect for setting the mood, but these sessions will still be valuable learning opportunities to help the orgasmic reflex along.

As you gradually learn the types of finger and hand movements as well as locations that elicit the most erotic feelings in you, begin to increase the speed and pressure of the movements to see if the erotic sensations increase and the clitoris gets harder and erect. We know it is difficult to do, but *don't think about orgasms!* Just concentrate on making those sensations even more pleasurable. Your short-term goal should be to become very knowledgeable about what pleases you. For some, long, slow, heavy pressured slides of the finger up and down the clitoris are best. For others it could be short, light flicks of the clitoris back and forth. Still other women are partial to rubbing with two fingers spread open on each side of the clitoris. Stimulating the clitoris was probably the basis for the expression: "Different strokes for different folks." So don't let anyone tell you how it "should" be done. Only *you* know that. (And, you have to know it well enough to teach your partner how best to stimulate you.)

Many women like to feel pressure inside their vaginas

while they are masturbating. Two or three fingers from the other hand may be placed inside the vagina while you are masturbating, or you might try one of the phallus-shaped vibrators mentioned in Chapter 5. (They are not very good for stimulation, but they can serve to give that sense of fullness in the vagina.) Or, you might want to use one of the latex dildos available. Many women find these dildos to be erotically satisfying for masturbation because of their smooth and supple texture. They are non-porous and easy to clean. They retain heat well, and you may want to warm them up first in a little heated water. (Caution: To avoid possible infection, never place a dildo, finger etc., first in your anus and then into your vagina.)

If even warm plastic leaves you cold, you might try a cucumber, as Betty Dodson suggests in her excellent book, *Sex for One*:

> An organic dildo can be made from a cucumber or zucchini (I have a friend who's crazy about wilted carrots too). A cucumber can be sculpted to size with a potato parer, but leave enough skin on the bottom for a handle so your lover won't slip away in the night. If you carve too close to the center seeds, the cucumber will go limp. Cucumbers are naturally moist and slippery and have been used in beauty creams for years.

Whatever you try should be done in the spirit of fun, adventure, and indulgence. *Don't think negatively!* If you think "O.K., I'll give it five or ten minutes, but nothing is going to happen," you can be assured that you will not have an orgasm. Say to yourself instead: "O.K., for the next few weeks I will massage and touch my clitoral area every single day with enthusiasm, fantasy, and imagination, and just let it happen sooner or later." Reducing expectations will increase your chances of success.

Remember, the bottom line is that masturbation and more masturbation is necessary to help you become orgasmic. Does this mean that every woman who is orgasmic has spent years and years masturbating? No! There are some women who apparently are naturally orgasmic and claim that they have never masturbated. For many others, nature needs your helping hand.

Religious Barriers to Masturbation

You may be reluctant to masturbate because of your early upbringing or religious training. You might even believe that it is wrong or sinful. What can you do about it? Well, there is really very little we can tell you in a book to help you overcome taboos, misinformation, and sometimes even downright cruel things said to children concerning masturbation. We would suggest that you see a pastoral counselor who understands the important role of sex in a happy marriage. If your objections to masturbation are not religious, you may want to see a psychologist. A well-informed religious minister or pastoral counselor will understand that sexual happiness is related to marital happiness and the general well-being of the family. Most religions today teach that sex for procreation does not have to be devoid of pleasure for the wife. Many ministers of the different religions will agree with the perspective of the sex therapist and give permission to use masturbatory activity for the duration of your therapeutic treatment. Later on, once you have learned to become orgasmic, you may be able to reach orgasm during intercourse and thus not encounter any religious conflict. Should you still need to stimulate yourself before or during intercourse, your clergyman is not likely to consider it masturbation—only a preparatory step in fulfilling conjugal responsibilities.

If you are a follower of a very strict clergyman, what you need to obtain from him is a temporary relaxation of the religious rules for *medical* reasons. This is not sinful self-indulgence but an exercise to achieve goals that will benefit the couple, her family, and her overall sense of self-esteem. As we discussed in our last book *Sex and Morality,* more and more clergy men and women recognize the importance and beauty of even non-procreational sex within a sanctified, loving relationship. The higher goals involved may allow the woman to be treated via masturbation without violation of conscience, but the religious reader may want to discuss this with her religious advisor.

Other Resistances to Masturbation

From the sex therapist's point of view, there is usually no way to help you become orgasmic without masturbation of the clitoris and clitoral area. Having your husband or partner touching you there will probably not result in orgasm if you are now non-orgasmic. The resistance you have about touching yourself is probably an extension of your resistance to bodily pleasure from any source. Remember, only *you* can allow the orgasm to occur; no one can "give" you an orgasm. Nor can you become orgasmic by way of psychotherapy, sex education, or a set of anatomical diagrams. All these may help prepare the way, just as we have been doing in this book, but ultimately it is up to your ability to masturbate and then transfer this pleasure-giving ability to your partner. Please don't fall into the trap of thinking: "If he really loved me, he would know what to do to help me have an orgasm," or even worse: "Maybe I can't have an orgasm because I really don't love him." The people who think this way are tragically allowing the sexual side of marriage to deteriorate even further.

Perhaps you grew up with the erroneous notion, made popular by Freud, that clitoral stimulation is infantile because it produces a "clitoral" orgasm rather than a "vaginal" one. You simply must rid your mind of the destructive view that a "healthy, mature" female's sexual stimulation—leading to orgasm—must come from vaginal penetration and thrusting of the penis. Freud's knowledge of female sexuality was only rudimentary, and we should not be bound by a myth that has belittled women who found great satisfaction and orgasms through clitoral masturbation. If Freud were looking over our shoulders as we write this, we are almost positive he would nod his head in approval of what we say in this matter.

Ellen's Complaint

If you have been following our exercise suggestions up to now, you probably are able to have orgasms when you want to as long as there is sufficient stimulation of the clitoris and surrounding area. But this doesn't always work out as smoothly as we would like it to. Recently, a client told us about a slight problem that she was having. She—let's call her Ellen—said that she was having no difficulty having an orgasm with the aid of her vibrator, but that when her partner performed oral sex on her, she did not always reach orgasm. Ellen also told us that she was not successful at bringing herself to orgasm when using only her fingers. Similarly, her partner was not able to bring her to orgasm with his fingers.

Of course, there are many possible explanations for the causes of these orgasmic slow-downs. The most likely one is that Ellen's partner is not pleasuring her correctly and sufficiently with his tongue and mouth or fingers. But if this were the case, Ellen should be able to bring herself to orgasm with her fingers once she had learned to do so through a vibrator. Not necessarily so. We have seen this situation before and believe that it has something to do with early negative associations concerning masturbation. We know that many children in the past were punished by their mothers who caught them masturbating—even at a very early age. (Unfortunately some parents still engage in this potentially harmful discipline.) Usually this occurs at an age far too young for the child to understand the reasons or morality behind the parent's objections. What we believe happens is that the child begins to sense that what he or she did—playing with the genitals—

must be wrong even though it feels good. Some of these children—unless this notion is overturned somewhere along their formative and adolescent years—may develop a problem preventing them from masturbating as they are growing up. At best they will feel uncomfortable or guilty when they do masturbate and much of the pleasure will be taken away.

We don't know if this is the case with Ellen. But if it is, then it is not too surprising that she cannot bring herself to orgasm with her fingers. Why then is she successful with her vibrator? Two possible explanations: first, since the vibrator is not part of her body and therefore represents a different situation from the childhood masturbation for which she might have been punished, there may not be the inhibition or guilt associated with her fingers; second, a good vibrator—used where it is most stimulating to Ellen—may be so intense that it overpowers any guilt feelings that might inhibit the orgasmic response.

What did we tell Ellen to do? The first thing we said was the most obvious. She must be more specific in telling her partner *exactly* how he should pleasure her orally or manually. In case this did not work after a few times, then she should use a method of *transference* to enable her to reach orgasm when stimulated only by her fingers or her partner. What do we mean by *transference?* It is transferring from a vibrator to her, or her partner's, fingers (or his tongue), the ability to reach orgasm.

Since in Ellen's case she is able to reach orgasm by using her vibrator, we told her to practice the following for a few times at home, preferably when she is without her partner. She was told to use her vibrator to bring her close to orgasm.

When she felt that it was almost beginning, Ellen was to switch over to her fingers to continue and complete the orgasm. We also reminded her of how important it is to pleasure herself in the vaginal area for a few moments afterward by using only her fingers. After a few sessions of this, Ellen was told to use her vibrator for only a moment or two and then to switch over to her fingers for the same time period—alternating between her fingers and the vibrator until she orgasms. Similarly, she was to do these exercises by alternating between her partner's fingers and her vibrator—and his tongue and the vibrator.

For many women, this is quite sufficient, but for some, and it turned out that Ellen was one of these women, a little more was needed. We also told her to pull out of her mental repertoire one of her favorite fantasies—or a new one as exciting as she could make it—and use this fantasy while she masturbates with her vibrator and fingers.

We have gone into length to explain the case of Ellen because we know that some people are worried that because they get so much pleasure from their vibrators, they may become dependent on them and not be able to achieve pleasure from an ordinary non-electronic finger or tongue. We doubt that this could happen but it is true that for some people the old "self-fulfilling prophecy" may come into play. For them, the fear that they have become too jaded by their vibrator's intensity and that they may not be satisfied by the old-fashioned ways is a real fear. If you should have such worries, take assurance from the situation of Ellen that it is no big deal to transfer the pleasure-inducing properties of the vibrator to the power of the fingers.

In the next chapter we shall use variations of these *transference* techniques to transfer the ability to bring yourself to orgasm through masturbation over to your lover so that he or she will be able to make you reach orgasm during coitus.

An Unusual Orgasmic Problem

For most women, being able to have orgasms through their own choosing and when they want to is sufficient. But there are some for whom this isn't enough. They have heard about women who are "multi-orgasmic" and would like to be like them. As far as the research literature goes, there is no mystery or secret about being multi-orgasmic, i.e., having one orgasm after another in a single sexual episode. It is a matter of desire, practice, and technique.

If you are able to have orgasms now and would like to become multi-orgasmic, here are a few things to remember. For one, many women report that after they reach orgasm, the clitoris becomes extremely sensitive—almost to the point of being painful if stimulation to the clitoris is maintained. In many cases, the woman pushes her partner's face away if he is performing cunnilingus on her, or she may push his hand away. This tends to signal to herself or her partner that she is finished with this sexual act. But since the arousal state for women is still very high at that point, she can easily have another orgasm, if she so desires.

What she should do to build up quickly to another orgasm is to alter the method of stimulation away from the clitoris itself to the surrounding areas, her nipples, or anus and quickly begin a new fantasy. Every once in a while she, or her partner, should briefly stimulate the clitoris to see if it is ready to receive the kind of pleasuring to allow her to come to orgasm. Of course, communication between you and your partner is vital for this to become successful. After a few sessions of this, you will find that you can be multi-orgasmic whenever you choose, with or without your partner. Of course, this is somewhat more difficult during coitus but it can be done with a little imagination and the willingness of the male to postpone his climax. How should he do that? Wait until the second half of this chapter!

Lost Orgasmic Ability

There are some women who have been orgasmic in the past, in sexual activity with a previous partner, but who no longer find themselves able to reach orgasm. Let's say that a woman is now in a loving relationship that she does not want to end. In this case, we would first have to know if she is able to bring herself to orgasm through masturbation. If not, we recommend the same exercises we prescribed for non-orgasmic women: reducing stress, creating a relaxed and conducive environment, developing fantasy skills, building erotic interest, and so forth.

Of course the problem may just lie with the incompetence of her partner. Believe it or not, there still are sexually incompetent and sexually illiterate adults out there. If she has a partner she loves who happens to be a boring lover, then she must become more of a sex educator than a sexual partner. The simplest thing to do is to take his hand and use his fingers as if they were her own and to bring herself to orgasm with her partner's fingers. After a few times, he will quickly learn to use his fingers and tongue in the way that will increase her erotic excitement to the point of orgasm.

Another way—and a very exciting way for most partners to learn—is to actually show him by lying back and telling him to closely observe you while you masturbate yourself to orgasm. (Allow yourself to make the sounds of pleasure you feel like making but try to also describe your activities so your partner can learn your favorite movements.)

Women have many different ways of being erotically stimulated to orgasm: fingers, hands, pillows, bedclothes, dildos, vibrators, massagers, tongues, big toes, penises, cucumbers, carrots, zucchini, water jets, bubbles, and so on. No one method is healthier, or more natural than another. It is only that some are more sophisticated, quicker, more convenient, cheaper, or more intense. But all paths lead to the same blissful destination. When it comes to wanting a partner to bring her to orgasm, however, a woman cannot expect her man to be a mind reader as to what is her preference for the moment and what is needed. She *must first* be fully aware of what brings her to orgasm before she can successfully communicate it to her partner. It doesn't really matter what methods or positions the couple use, as long as she is satisfied with her orgasm and he is happy with what he is doing.

We have often heard about men who put pressure on their sexual partners to have orgasm during intercourse. For some women, due to anatomical, psychological, or situational reasons, this is not an attainable goal. The important thing for men to realize is that it is not so much whether the orgasm occurs during penetration but rather that the woman has a satisfying orgasm. Certainly, there is no medical *value* attached to the woman having the orgasm during penetration, since it is not more likely to induce conception (if she is trying to have a baby). For man or woman the sex act is not more "complete" if the woman's orgasm occurs when the penis is penetrating. Nor is orgasm during coitus more likely to provide the satisfactory resolution feeling of well-being than any other way of providing the orgasm.

There are also some people who still believe that "simultaneous orgasm" is the ultimate goal of sexual intercourse. It is a pity that so many men and women felt inadequate in the past because they could not achieve this sexual goal during coitus as deemed "ideal" by that well-intentioned but misguided grand-daddy of sex manuals: *Ideal Marriage* by Theodore Van de Velde. While there is nothing abnormal about such a goal, be aware that for the reasons we have given above, it may not be achievable and even if it is, many men and women say that when this happens they cannot fully appreciate the beauty of the orgasm in their partners because they are so involved with their own sensations.

Flat Moments

We said earlier, in Chapter 2, that some women experience a flat moment before the orgasmic response where it looks as if nothing is going to happen. This could lead to a woman thinking that nothing else is going to happen, and so she "turns herself off." If this happens to you while practicing the masturbation exercises, you can get past it by continuing. It may be as simple as that. At that moment you must continue and even *increase* the stimulation of the clitoris and the clitoral area until new heights of sensation are reached. For some women, this "quiet before the storm" is a necessary prelude to the orgasmic response. In many ways, this is like a meditative state that nature builds into women so that they can clear the "chatter in the head" and focus on the developing sensations to come in the impending orgasm. But if you fill your head with anxieties, doubts, and distractions instead, the sensation of the moment may be lost—and so the orgasm. One may also look at the "flat moment" in a positive way as the point in the orgasmic process where you consciously remove your thinking from the process and allow your bodily sensation to take over. View this momentary lack of sensation as the heralding of new and higher sensations. This is the time for you to focus solely on the sensations produced by a simple fantasy of your clitoris being stimulated by the hand, tongue, or penis of the person you most desire intimacy with at that moment. Latch on to that scene and stay with it, while increasing the intensity of your stimulation for a few minutes longer in order to reach the high point.

Retarded Orgasm

There are some women who complain that they are only able to have orgasms after a lengthy session of either self-stimulation or with much help of a partner. To them, sex has become work and thus it detracts from the sense of satisfaction after orgasm. They would enjoy the entire experience more (and so would their partners, who often have to do most of the "work") if they could only reach orgasm more quickly. All this "hard work" is fairly easy to circumvent *if* you have done what we have told you to do throughout this book, *and* you rule out medication or alcohol and you remember to use those fantasies that seem to have worked best for you in the past. Vary the setting, the mood, the scents, the strokes, and so forth until you find the right combination that works best for you. Introduce some fun into your sex life. Laughter is one of the best known stress-reducers, and it may be underlying stress that helps delay the orgasm. In any case, take control, *don't complain,* and make a better sex life happen.

Pain

As we indicated back in Chapter 2, a woman might feel pain upon penetration and after penetration. Again, any pain should be taken very seriously, and consultation with a gynecologist is in order. However, if there is nothing physically wrong with your vagina, then you may try some of our suggestions. If the pain persists, then please see a medical specialist in order to be treated.

The most likely source of pain for the woman, whether upon entrance of the penis or even for some time after, is the lack of lubrication. How does this come about? Here, a knowledge of the causes determines the ways in which you can eliminate the pain. The lack of lubrication may result from the use of antihistamines or other medications that work, in part, by drying up the mucus in the sinus area. For some women, they may have a more general effect including that of inhibiting the vaginal lubrication. If your lack of vaginal lubrication occurs when you have been taking some kind of medication, ask your physician about it and have him suggest alternative medications that don't have this effect upon you.

If the lack of lubrication stems from insufficient physical or erotic stimulation, go back to the earlier chapters in this book and practice your erotic skills. Remember the answer to the question asked by the visitor to New York City: "How do you get to Carnegie Hall?" The answer: "Practice, practice, practice!"

Whether your lack of stimulation has to do with a temporary condition or you usually do not lubricate sufficiently, use a good lubricant such as K-Y Jelly. Some women prefer the feeling of Vaseline, which is O.K. as long as you are not using a diaphragm or condom. (A petroleum jelly, such as Vaseline, can weaken the materials in those birth control devices.)

If the lack of lubrication is due to your 60-second husband or lover, then you must take on the role of educator and make him sexually literate about *your entire* body. It may not be that he is selfish or doesn't care. We find that even in this day and age, there are many men who just don't know anything about their wives' sexual responses. This is particularly true where the wife has sometimes pretended or exaggerated her passion in order to make him feel better. Such deception only lets the husband think that whatever he is doing must be right. Don't expect miracles of knowledge by osmosis or revelation in sexual matters. Nature does not provide us with a textbook, and a man can only learn about a woman's sexuality from his lover. So talk to him and tell him exactly what you want. Take his hand and show him, if necessary.

Vaginismus

Some women experience pain upon penetration because the vaginal muscles have tightened up so much that the opening becomes too narrow for the penis to enter comfortably. What can you do if you think you have this type of problem? First, be on the safe side and check with a gynecologist to make sure there is nothing physically wrong. You don't want to undertake sex therapy for a problem that should be corrected medically. But if there is nothing physically wrong, don't necessarily see a clinical psychologist or psychiatrist before trying a *dilator* on yourself. These may be purchased on the prescription of your physician, who will suggest the correct sizes, through some medical supply houses, or through adult outlets. They vary in length from a few inches to about seven inches, and their circumferences also vary from about the thickness of a finger to those thicker than a penis. Sometimes, smaller size *dildos* may be used as a dilator if you start with the smallest size.

Whichever you use, first apply a lot of lubrication (and don't forget the fantasies). Place your finger inside first, to get your vagina accustomed to the feel of something inside. After a few minutes, when you feel comfortable with your finger, you can remove it, add more lubrication, and very gently slide the dilator inside. If there appears to be strong resistance, slide it in ever so slowly to make sure you experience no pain. By the way, don't confuse those dilators that look like erect penises with the kind of dilator or speculum that is used by a gynecologist for the internal vaginal examination. The medical type spreads the muscles open with a little pressure from the doctor, while the dilators we are talking about relax the muscles and allow the vagina to accept insertions.

Lack of Sexual Desire

Now, what do you do if you are interested in sex, you have a loving, significant other, you are able to lubricate and there is no pain on penetration—you want to have sex, but it seems that you just don't have the "horniness" (the sense of sexual urgency), that you once had or think you should have? Instead, you feel: "Sex—I can take it or leave it." You have no aversion to sex, but no real desire for it either. First, you should review our previous chapters about building your erotic interest in sex and reducing any stress that may inhibit your sexual desires. If you feel that you have done all you could do to build desire, that you are not angry at your partner, and that you are not using any medications that may lower the libido (such as some fungicides, glaucoma medications, or cough medicines), then you probably have some interpersonal relationship problems or even more deeply rooted problems that should be evaluated by a marriage counselor or psychologist.

Only you can get a feel for the underlying source of the problem—whether it is anger at the partner, concern about the permanency of the relationship, money, disappointments, unrealistic expectations, or whatever. If you sometimes get a sense that these are the real issues that are turning you off, you can bring this up to your partner and say: "Let's fight these out in the living room rather than in bed." It also may help if you take an "inventory" of your marital strengths and weaknesses. On one side of a sheet of paper place all those things that you are happy about in your relationship; on the other side, write down all the negative aspects of the relationship. Candidly discuss the negative points with your partner, but also stress the good points in the relationship so that these strengths can help the two of you overcome the difficulties as you perceive them.

More often than not, the lack of sexual desire is related to some problem in the emotional life that exists between the couple or is in some manner situational, that is, due to one or more of the issues we mentioned in Chapter 2. They are so important in negatively affecting our sex lives that we should examine them again at this point:

- *Stress from work, parenting, money shortages, etc.*
- *Fear of becoming pregnant*
- *Lack of erotic and sensual practice*
  Not enough practice in pleasuring the body
- *Fear of sexual fantasizing and revealing the subconscious*
  Homosexual, incestuous, and other forbidden images come to mind

- *Problems with your partner*
  Poor hygiene, weight gain, sexual illiteracy, anger
- *Medications, alcohol, and other drugs*
  Over-the-counter medications like cold preparations, excessive drinking, opiates, "downers," and others
- *Changing male and female roles*
  Coping with the more assertive woman, equality in marriage, and the elimination of the double standard
- *Aversion to genitalia*
  Unconscious thoughts about the vagina or penis being "dirty," "smelly," or "dangerous"
- *Sexual abuse as a child or adult*
  Incest, rape, sexual molestation, or psychosexual abuse
- *Poor self-image*
  Growing up with verbal abuse by parents: "We hope you will be lucky enough to find some man who will marry you."
- *Boredom*
  You've done it all, "Is that all there is, my friend?"

Stress

If you have carefully read this book and practiced our suggestions, you have gained valuable methods to cope with the stress factors in your life. No matter how much you have succeeded in reducing stress, as we've advocated, everyone will continue to experience some stress in his or her life. But not everyone allows it to interfere with his or her sex life. Those who don't allow stress to adversely affect them are those who have acknowledged the reality of stress and have *taken charge* by finding alternatives to stressful situations. Stress-reducing solutions often lie in financial counseling, parenting groups, and vocational counseling. If you feel there is little you can do to avoid your stressful situations by relying on these external supports, you can concentrate on those methods we suggested earlier such as meditation to help prevent stress from harming you and your sex life. If you still find that you can't cope with stress on your own, you might try to consult with a stress-reduction expert at a clinic that specializes in this kind of therapy. Your physician should be able to help you, or you might inquire at a pain clinic in a hospital near you. Most pain clinics are very knowledge about stress-reduction techniques and have contact with other clinics or programs that specialize in stress reduction. It is most desirable if you can learn to manage the stress on your own through developing your stress-reducing skills because it will have a spin-off in the way that you manage the rest of your life. But if you can't, then seek professional help.

Fear of Pregnancy

If the fear of pregnancy is producing your situational lack of desire, the solutions depend on whether or not your religion places any restrictions on various methods of contraception. If there is no problem with religious regulations, then your gynecologist will suggest the method best suited to you and your physical condition. If there is still a deep-set pervasive anxiety about the pill, diaphragm, or condom not working, then try two methods of contraception at the same time. For example, use a diaphragm while your husband uses a condom. There are more women who play it doubly safe than you think. If this is necessary to give you peace of mind, so what? There is nothing strange about both the man and the woman using contraceptives at the same time. If the fear still persists to the point of inhibiting your erotic responses or your desire for sex, then you should consult with a psychologist. You have to rule out the possibility that this fear is the result of not wanting a child in the particular relationship in which you find yourself—or there may be some deeper causes for the fear.

An extreme fear of becoming pregnant may seem outrageous to some people, but there are many women who see pregnancy as catastrophic for them because of their particular life situation at the time. While we respect the rights and duty of any religion to condemn and prohibit abortion for its adherents, we have encountered women who become pregnant and who desperately seek an abortion. Because they will take any risk to their own lives, a safe, legal abortion by a qualified doctor must remain an option for those women whose religious convictions allow one. We are not for abortion as a contraceptive measure, and we view abortion as a serious matter and one of last resort. We believe this to be true whether the pregnancy is due to contraceptive failure, date rape, abandonment by the father, seduction of a teenager by an adult, or whatever situation was involved in the pregnancy. To our knowledge, the decision to have an abortion was never taken lightly by women and almost always occurred where there was no reasonable alternative.

If there is a religious prohibition against artificial contraception, you may still be able to successfully avoid an unwanted pregnancy with abstinence during the fertile period of your menstrual cycle. You can learn how to determine these fertile days from your gynecologist. Many people refer to this as the rhythm or "natural" method.

Lack of Erotic Practice

What can you do if you have tried our previous chapters' advice about shower massagers, bubble baths, candlelight, erotic fantasizing, sex breaks and all the rest, and you still have no desire for sex? First of all, you have to be honest with yourself about the extent to which you practiced, and honest about the possible changes for the better that you noticed. How much did you practice? Did you give it just ten minutes for three days or did you really try it every day for three months? Were you totally aware of any physical or psychological sensations that were different—for example, nipples becoming erect when you touched your breasts. If they never reacted before it indicates that you were moving in the right direction. Maybe you only need more time. Give yourself a few more weeks to become even more sensitive to slight changes in your erotic responses and attitudes and what it was that precipitated these changes. Once you learn this you can increase the frequency of the types of activity that bring on these responses. If there is really no change that you can see, and your desires have not at all increased, then you probably should consult with a psychologist to determine if the problems are on a deeper level than just lack of erotic practice.

Fear of Sexual Fantasizing and Revealing the Subconscious

How do people handle those spontaneous images and thoughts of sex acts they were taught were forbidden—homosexuality, incest, exhibitionism, etc.—which sometimes come to mind and may cause a temporary loss of sexual desire? We know that it is very difficult, probably impossible, to prevent all thoughts like these from coming to mind now and then. If you should be bothered by such thoughts, remember that the thought is not the reality. Spontaneous fantasies of all sorts are perfectly normal and all people have them. The real issue is whether you allow these thoughts to inhibit or cripple your sexual desires and behavior. There is certainly nothing wrong with merely having these thoughts.

In a sense, you have to learn to give yourself permission to have these fantasies, knowing that this is all there is to it and that you will never act upon them or reveal them to anyone. Now, if the thoughts are very threatening to you, you might try to redirect the spontaneous fantasy or thought when it arises by immediately replacing it with a safe image and repeat the safe image in your mind, over and over, until the forbidden thought is gone. This is similar to using a mantra during meditation. Thus, if you have learned how to reduce stress by using the "relaxation response" of Dr. Herbert Benson discussed in an earlier chapter, you can now apply the same technique to eliminate, for the moment, these unwanted sexual thoughts.

It is important to understand that not all spontaneous fantasies mean what you think they mean. For many people, these threatening thoughts are similar to the "wishes" of small children who say to their parents: I hate you, I wish you were dead. We know that these "wishes" are not what the child really means, but they represent a childish inability to express the real nature of the problem and feelings as perceived by the child. In a sense, the child does not know how to communicate its true feelings and so an extreme image comes out as a substitute. Similarly, some adults may not be able to express their love for a friend or relative and so this love feeling emerges in a thought that some people associate with love: sex. This may also be true of incestuous feelings where the very strong feelings of love get confused with sexual images. Why does this sometimes happen? We believe that it may be due to a confusion of words and concepts that exists in our language. How often have we heard the word "love" used when the speaker really means a sexual act? We hear it so often in popular music lyrics and everyday talk: "Love me tonight as you never have before" or "Did you ever make love to her?" While not everybody is confused about the differences between love and sex, there is an unconscious danger in the interchangeability of the two. When we become aware of how often we may confuse love with lust, we may then stop having these unwanted thoughts.

If you have tried all of our suggestions and are still troubled by these thoughts, we think it would be wise to consult with a professional in this area who will be able to help you sort out the reasons behind your thoughts.

Problems with Your Partner

Poor Hygiene

One of the most common problems we hear about is an embarrassing one for many men and women to talk about. This has to do with unwanted odors that turn some people off from their sexual desires. Because one tends to become accustomed to one's own body odors and because our own odors don't usually emanate near our own noses, people are often unaware of such offenses until their spouses or significant others tell them about it. For example, some people are careless about cleaning themselves properly after they go to the bathroom, about washing themselves all over the body when in the shower, or about brushing their teeth. In some cases, it might be ulcers, digestive problems, or tooth or gum decay that is causing the problem. For women, proper cleaning of the vaginal area should result in no unpleasant odor for her lover, but many women may not be aware of the odors at the early stages of yeast infections or other problems. Unfortunately, many men assume that the vagina of a woman naturally "smells" and are uncomfortable about telling their loved ones about it.

Now, before you think we are advocating sterilizing the skin before two people have sex, we are also aware that many people over-react to even the slightest odors, having been brought up to have very negative feelings about body odors. When they were very young they may have been somewhat harshly taught to control odors from different parts of the body so that no one should notice them. Consequently, when they are grown up and smell these odors on someone else, it brings to mind an image of someone not controlling "dirty" odors. They feel that these odors should not be present in an interpersonal situation, even between a husband and wife. Remember, there is a certain amount of natural odors that is present even with proper hygiene. There are even some odors—sweat for example—that may actually turn people on sexually. So, before you rush to take a shower each and every time you want to have sex, you really should discuss these issues with your partner.

There are also situations involving odors and loss of desire that are due to more serious issues. We are referring, for example, to women who have been sexually or physically abused by their drunken fathers when they were young. Consequently, the smell of alcoholic drinks on the breath of even a very loving husband may bring back negative memories and a very strong aversion to intimacy associated with these odors. Because many women with these childhood experiences have suppressed their memories of the events, they may just react negatively toward their husbands without knowing why. These women should see a psychologist because unless the problem is dealt with, it will have an increasingly negative impact on the relationship. But even in these cases, try discussing these problems first. It may be that just bringing it out in the open will help.

Weight Gain

What about being turned off by your own, or a lover's weight gain? Here we have to be careful not to get trapped by media-created images of what a man or woman should look like. If we believe that a "healthy" woman should have a body like Cher or Jane Fonda, and a healthy man should look like Tom Selleck or Don Johnson, then we could become ashamed of our own looks or those of our partners. Remember, you can have fantastic sex and have the strongest sex drive even if you look like "Jack Spratt who ate no fat" or "his wife who ate no lean." Not only in the Middle Ages were "sanftig" (soft, chubby) women most desirable but even in the Twentieth Century, a heavier man was considered more prosperous and successful because it indicated that he had the money to eat well. Among many immigrants to this country, having a healthy child meant having a "chubby" child because people believed that fat was healthier and more attractive than thin. A trimmer, firmer body should be desired because it is healthier for you, but not because it has become fashionable. If your body weight, or that of your spouse, gets so high that it physically interferes with your having sex, that is another matter. That kind of obesity should be medically treated as soon as possible. If it is just a slight weight gain on the part of your spouse, this should not affect your sexual desires—unless you are using this as an excuse for something more seriously wrong with your marriage. Certainly discuss this with your spouse and if it appears that your lack of desire is not due to a correctable weight problem but more serious aspects in the relationship, then see a relationship or marital counselor.

Sexual Illiteracy

Even in the 1990s, we still see women who have "turned off" their sexual desires because of the sexual incompetence of their mates. Their husbands were sexually illiterate for all their years of marriage, not realizing that their wives' clitorises and other areas must be stimulated and successfully aroused before penetration. For their part, the wives did not masturbate to help stimulate themselves. And so they fell into a pattern of boring sexual passivity, thinking that there must be something wrong with their sexual responsiveness.

When a man thinks that all he has to do to satisfy a woman is to enter her and pump away, then he is clearly a sexual illiterate. Unfortunately, some women feed into their husbands' illiteracy by pretending with moans and groans to be enjoying the one-way sex. Sometimes they even pretend to have an orgasm because they don't want to hurt the feelings of the men they love. These women may feel very dutiful and even considerate, but they are needlessly frustrated. If you are in this kind of situation, you must first take charge of your own stimulation through the various techniques described in this book. Then you must help your husband in a gentle, non-threatening way by reading this book together and discussing the various things you would like him to do to you.

Anger

Sometimes, people are not aware that they are angry at their partners. There are people who seem to be constantly angry, not only at their spouses but at everyone and everything. When you talk to them you find that there isn't one particular thing that makes them angry—something that might easily be changed or avoided—but it appears to be life itself. Well, it is pretty hard to retain much sexual desire for others when you are filled with such feelings of anger. If you sense this anger in yourself, or if others point it out to you, then you must do something about it. You can't have good sex with a "chip on your shoulder." Even if you try the auto-erotic exercises we have talked about earlier, you will only bring this anger to your own body. If the stress-reduction exercises do not have a significant impact upon your feelings and subsequent sexual desires, then you must seek the services of a clinical psychologist.

Medications, Alcohol, and Other Drugs

As we have mentioned, different kinds of over-the-counter and prescription medications, can lower the libido, that is lowering or even temporarily eliminating sexual desire. Some, like hypertension medications, may even cause temporary impotence for a man. Some medications may "dry up" the woman so that she does not lubricate properly, making intercourse unpleasant or painful. This complicated matter should be discussed with your physician, since there are usually alternative medications without these side effects. Even innocuous over-the-counter medicines may cause sexual functioning problems in ways you might not suspect. For example, many cough medicines or antihistamines may make you drowsy enough to prefer a bed for sleeping rather than for good sex. Use your common sense and read the small print on any medications, even the non-prescription ones. Always ask your pharmacist or physician to tell you about the possible side effects of prescription medications. If it makes you too drowsy "to handle heavy machinery," you may be too drowsy for the delicate machinery of the genitalia and libido.

In any case, if you experience any sudden change in your sexual desires or normal sexual functioning after taking a new medication, immediately contact your doctor as you should after any side effect from a medication. The same is true if you "self-medicate," that is, decide on your own what you believe your illness or condition to be and find an over-the-counter medication for it. If you have *any* negative reaction from *any* medicine, tell your doctor immediately.

Another drug, which we sometimes forget is a drug, that may also decrease the libido or cause temporary impotence is alcohol. The messages about alcohol are often confusing because, on the one hand, we often hear, and rightly so, that having a glass or two of wine can relax a person to more easily permit and build up sexual desires. On the other hand, "too much" alcohol has just the opposite effect on both men and women. The key phrase here is too much. Keep in mind that alcohol, an intoxicant, works like a sedative. It slows down the responses and sensitivity of nerve endings, including those related to sexual pleasure and performance. So, be careful and don't drink yourself out of your pleasure.

Changing Male and Female Roles

Although we already discussed the major issues involved in the sexual relationship as a consequence of the changes in male and female roles, we would like to re-emphasize these implications for the bedroom. The fact is that many men are still confused and anxious about the new assertiveness of women that is rapidly becoming institutionalized in our society. We have seen that, for some men and women, this anxiety may be translated into a decrease or even temporary loss of the usual sexual desires. (See our discussion in the last chapter: "The Working Woman and Changing Sex Roles.") We must add here that these larger societal changes do have impact on relationships. Too many men and women who resist these changes blame their spouse or lover for causing this discomfort and behaving differently than the partner they had chosen to live with. These men and women have to come to grips with the reality that profound changes from the outside do affect life in the living room *and* the bedroom. The old ways of relating to one another, based on what life was like when we were growing up, must be brought up to date and re-evaluated.

Whatever the male/female tensions may be in your relationship, they are bound to have an impact in the bedroom. The old stereotypical norm—that the husband is the breadwinner—went hand in hand with the notion that the man provides the initiative for sex and that the husband has a "right" to demand sexual gratification. Today, more and more women are equal "breadwinners." Because they feel sexually equal to their husbands, they are less inhibited about showing their sexual equality and will more frequently take the initiative. In some cases, their newly found multi-orgasmic potential may even threaten a spouse with very old-fashioned ideas about female sexuality.

It is understandable that men and women are often confused these days, because there are parental role models that seem to be inconsistent with today's world—and we certainly don't, and never did, have parental role models for sexual behavior. If one looks to television for some sort of guidelines or models—as many people unconsciously do—it is very confusing. While TV women are not as passive with their husbands as before, most TV spouses are not true "equals." When the male is the aggressor, in business and sex, he is reinforcing an old "macho" stereotype. When we see the female as aggressor, in business or sex, she is often portrayed as a manipulative bitch. Hollywood and TV are still not very fair to women these days.

We don't have any easy solution to these problems especially during this era of changes. But be aware that these problems are real and affect men and women in their sexual and emotional relationships. At least try to reduce the stress through the means we suggested earlier and bring these discomforts out in the open. If your or your spouse's changing role seems to be making you uncomfortable, discuss it openly—but not in bed. There is nothing to be ashamed of if you wish the old sex roles had not changed, but don't take it out on your spouse because they have.

Aversion to Genitalia

Some people have great anxiety and can even experience a phobic or panic reaction when touching or putting their faces near their partners' genitals. In other cases, having one's genitals touched or engaging in coitus brings on similar reactions. In these cases of extreme fear or disgust we recommend a sex therapist who is also a physician or a psychiatrist who is qualified to treat this complex problem with the appropriate medications and psychotherapy. Dr. Helen Singer Kaplan has pioneered work in this type of problem and has written a book called *Sexual Aversion, Sexual Phobias, and Panic Disorder.* The problem is serious but treatable.

Sexual Abuse as a Child or Adult

This is another serious problem that we are learning more about each day. Many more people than we were aware of apparently had been sexually abused when they were very young. It should come as no surprise that this kind of terrible experience endured by a young girl or boy will have a negative effect upon the victim's adult sexual functioning. Because of the complicated nature of this problem it is best if a clinical psychologist deals with these patients. If he or she thinks that sex therapy, as an adjunct to psychotherapy, might also help, then work with the suggestions in this book or see a sex therapist. As with the previous discussion, this is not a hopeless problem, but don't count on "time" to heal wounds this deep. Get professional help.

Poor Self-Image

One major group of problems seems to result from people acting out the "script" that was written for them many years ago. That is, they got married, had a loving spouse, had lovely children, but now feel that there was nothing special that they did with their lives. They carried out their parental script for what a "good girl" should do, but somehow they just don't feel very good about themselves. These women, who some people describe as having "low self-esteem," are often that way because they were put down by their mothers or fathers when they were young. They were made to feel that they were really nobody special, and that marriage and family is the best that they could do. In many cases, their parents used to voice doubts that they would even get married.

Sometimes, these people have negative feelings about themselves reinforced by their spouses, friends, acquaintances, or superiors at work. We know people with low self-esteem who create a "self-fulfilling prophecy" in daily interactions with other people. They start the day feeling negative about themselves, project those feelings to everyone around them, and, in some sense, *force* others to treat them as if they didn't count for much in this world. All these negative feelings must stop—and not only because it is bound to affect your sexual desire but also because you have a *right* to feel good about yourself. How do you do this?

There are many ways to think more positively about yourself and many books on the subject of positive thinking. Some methods work for some people and others work for other people. Try to find a self-help book that might work for you and, if necessary, seek some professional help to overcome any destructive patterns of thinking. Develop some skills or hobbies that you enjoy and can be good at. You might even discover you have a talent for playing the piano, painting, or choral singing. Most important of all: Do something about the people who put you down. If they are acquaintances, drop them. If they are friends, have a candid talk with them about the situation because, as we said earlier, with friends like these, who needs enemies? If your spouse is putting you down, run, don't walk, to a marriage counselor and drag your spouse with you before you allow what is good in your marriage to deteriorate. In other words: *Don't complain.* Stand up for yourself and take control of your life, even if it means confronting the people closest to you!

Boredom

We are not now referring to sexual boredom, because Chapters 4, 5, and 6 should be consulted if you are still sexually bored. Rather, we mean a general *ennui* or boredom in one's life that sometimes results in a lack of sexual desire or interest. Boredom, too, is *your* responsibility. People don't make you bored. And certainly life is not boring, but *you* can make life boring for yourself. No one has to be bored. You can take some time out of your week, no matter how busy you are, and do interesting and exciting things, even on a voluntary basis. Look around—there are political organizations that can use you, or hospitals, day-care centers, museums, the auxiliary police, the volunteer fire department, or whatever.

Sometimes, boredom comes with having too much time on one's hands. That is, a couple is retired or one spouse outlives the other but is still very healthy. But what should they do to fill large amounts of time? Think of some big, exciting changes. For example, consider joining a voluntary group in your area. Dedicated volunteers have a different walk about them. You can see these people in the street. They have what the French call a *raison d'être,* a "reason for being." They seem more alive than the people around them, and we will bet that they have happier sex lives as well. Everybody needs goals and interests in life so that life can be constantly challenging, enabling you to grow and expand your horizons and experiences. This is true of all ages, but particularly so as you get older.

Challenges and goals are "built in" for younger people as they try to establish themselves in the world and raise a happy and healthy family. But as you achieve these necessary goals, and security seems on the way, you have time to think about yourself and reflect on what you have accomplished with your life. We should all remember the words of the great Rabbi Hillel: "If I am not for myself, who will be for me? If I am only for myself, then what am I? If not now, when?" You need new worlds to conquer to revitalize the *joie de vivre* that is so necessary for all adults who want emotionally happy and satisfying lives. While it may be true that an empty emotional and social life probably indicates a bad sex life, it is also true that a strong sex drive and good sex life can't fill an otherwise empty life. So go out there and chase a long-postponed dream. And, rest assured that as you increase your *joie de vivre* you will notice a marked increase in your sexual desires. If boredom had been instrumental in turning down your libido, your new passion for that ideal or hobby should spill over to your bedroom.

Getting Older

As we said back in Chapter 2, one of the most prevalent sexual myths is the one that men and women lose their sexual drives and ability to perform as they get older. Total nonsense! For some women, orgasms may become more intense as they get on in years, while for others the intensity may remain the same or even decline a bit. But certainly if you were orgasmic, you will still be able to bring on this wonderful sensation by yourself or with the help of others. And even if you never had orgasms, it is never too late to begin!

We would recommend that the older woman place a greater emphasis upon lubrication, because that is frequently lessened with age. If a younger woman does not lubricate sufficiently when she wants to have sex, it usually means that she has not been sufficiently stimulated, by herself or her partner and that she is not ready for intercourse. But when an older woman does not lubricate, it may mean that the physiology of aging just doesn't permit her to lubricate as much as she needs. It doesn't mean that her libido has changed or that she is not desirous of sex.

The treatment for reduced lubrication involves two things. First: increased erotic stimulation and even a little fantasy. Second: use a good lubricant such as K-Y jelly. Even for masturbation, we would recommend that the older woman use a good lubricant, and it is always a good idea for her to use some during intercourse to avoid any pain.

Another problem we sometimes see in the older woman is one that is not really her problem but one imposed upon her by TV, movies, advertising, and so forth. These media put so much emphasis upon youth and the so-called "beautiful people," that they make many older women think that they are no longer attractive, especially sexually, to their husbands or to any other men. But we are only as old or as attractive as we feel. Many of the activities suggested here will make you feel and be more desirable because they put you in touch with your capacity for desire and pleasure. Inactivity is the enemy for people of all ages. The more active you become with desirable interests, the more desirable and interesting you will be.

There are some women, however, in whom a loss of sexual desire may be due to hormonal changes. Women who notice a sharp drop in their libidos should discuss this with a physician. If it turns out that your loss of desire is partly or mainly psychological, then, you should follow the kinds of activities we have suggested throughout this book. Whatever hormonal components of the loss of desire your physician discovers are, of course, for medical personnel to treat. All this assumes that you have a comfortable relationship with your physician so that you can freely discuss your lack of sexual desire. But for many women, it is not that easy to discuss this topic. If you are one of these women, what should you do? When you go to your physician, don't wait for the physician to begin the discussion of sex, particularly if it is a male physician. Even though you may have some difficulty talking about sex, keep in mind that your physician, especially if he came from the same background as yours probably has the same hang-ups about discussing sex comfortably as most people seem to. Many physicians have had little training in human sexuality at medical school, so you will have to ask the right questions. If your physician cannot give you a satisfactory answer to your sex questions, he should refer you to someone. So, don't wait for your physician to take the initiative in asking you about any changes in your sex drive— you must bring the subject up at first notice. Just as we say, *Don't Complain*, we now say *Don't Wait!*

Remember, coping with stress, being more erotically oriented, pleasuring your body, learning to turn yourself on, and the importance of masturbation are not just for young people. These are some of the ways, along with love and commitment and caring, for all of us to have more satisfying sexual enjoyment for the rest of our lives.

Using Your PC

No, we don't mean using your *personal computer.* We mean your *pubococcygeal* muscle, sometimes called the "PC" muscle and even the "Love" muscle by some writers. The main muscle in the pelvic area, the more firmly toned it is, the more a woman may avoid urinary stress and other problems in the pelvic area. Reported research findings on this muscle also establish that women seem to enjoy sex more and appear to be more likely to have orgasms when it is in good shape. We think that women should exercise this important muscle as they do other muscles in their body in order to stay fit.

Certainly, as in all other exercise programs, check with your physician first to see if you have any other problems that might be present.

It is fairly easy to identify the PC muscle. It is the muscle that you use when you want to cut off the flow of urine at will. Another way you can identify this muscle is to lie on your back, and place one of your fingers about two inches inside of your vagina. Then contract the muscles in your vaginal area just as if you wanted to stop the flow of urine. You will feel the pubococcygeal muscle tighten around your finger. Hold it there, tightly, for a few seconds. Then relax. These two motions of tightening and relaxing are essentially all you have to do to strengthen this important muscle. It will come in handy when you and your partner want to experiment with somewhat different sensations during intercourse. Try this exercise once or twice a day for a few minutes at a time. Each time you tighten the muscle, hold it tight for 5 or 6 seconds, then slowly and completely relax the muscle. After a few seconds, repeat the contraction and relaxing of the muscle. After a few weeks, you might want to hold the contraction for about 10 seconds or more. We can't promise that toning up this muscle will definitely increase your likelihood to have orgasms or the frequency or intensity of orgasms, but at least you can use this new strength for an interesting variation during intercourse.

During coitus with the woman on top, instead of moving the body up and down or forward and back, sit still and contract the PC muscle around the penis in such a way as if you were drawing the penis deeper into the vagina. After a few seconds, slowly relax and repeat the cycle. You should soon get into a rhythm of contraction and relaxation that approximates the increasing movement in most instances of intercourse. (Knowledge of this skill was brought back by many servicemen who had experienced this with Asian women, who seemed to be better *trained* at sexual pleasuring than most women in Western culture.) You can increase the speed of these contractions until the man ejaculates. While doing this, he can stimulate your clitoris with his fingers or with a vibrator to bring you to orgasm.

A side benefit of these exercises and of this particular sexual position is that when your male lover is unusually tired or seems to have more difficulty getting an erection than when he was younger, you can sit on top of him, stuff his penis inside of you and stimulate his penis to erection with these contractions. Many men report that this experience is fantastic!

And Speaking of Men . . .

As we have suggested for the women, you have to learn how to deal with problems on your own before you can work on any sexual problems or dissatisfactions during intercourse. Just as a woman should learn to take responsibility and bring herself to orgasm before involving someone else in the therapeutic process, a man too should gain control over whatever his problem is before taking that difficulty to bed. We know that it is more pleasurable to have a loved one help you at a time of need and it feels more mechanical when you do these exercises by yourself, but the nature of sex problems is such that it is best you don't run the risk of a sexual letdown in front of another person. Be patient and wait until the next chapter.

But before we begin: Did you follow our program of erotic exercises? That is, did you practice your erotic fantasy skill development, appreciate your body's sensuality more, think more erotically, eliminate or change any medications, illicit drugs, or alcohol that might interfere, and so forth? Please, do all this first *before* you work on your specific problem. You may be pleasantly surprised to learn that if you faithfully do all these things, *you will no longer have a problem.* This is even more true for men than for women because these factors seem to impact more on the sexual *functioning* of men.

Premature Ejaculation

Let's begin with the most common complaint: premature ejaculation. As we said in Chapter 3, any dissatisfaction with the length of time from the point of arousal to the point of ejaculation may be classified under this condition. Usually, it is the man himself who is dissatisfied with his inability to delay ejaculation, but sometimes it is only his partner who is unhappy. Even if the man wants to control his ejaculation only to please his partner, the solutions to the problem are the same.

Because the male usually has to have an erection before ejaculation, bringing on that erection is the first order of business. How he does that will vary. It is very important that he learns to control his erections as well as his ejaculations. He should practice the different kinds of erotic stimulation we have talked about throughout this book, learning which fantasies and auto-erotic techniques will best bring him to an erection. Once he has an erection, however, *he should not continue to fantasize.* Instead, he should concentrate on the sensations that occur as he strokes his penis. He must learn to identify the premonitory sensation. The premonitory sensation is what you feel at that moment before the point of no return—before the ejaculation is inevitable. Some therapists call this the "moment of inevitability." Once that threshhold has passed, it is too late to delay the ejaculation which occurs beyond your control. It is only when you learn to recognize the sensations that occur *before* this moment that you can learn to control the ejaculation.

After slowly masturbating a few times and concentrating on the sensations immediately preceding ejaculation, you will soon learn to recognize that premonitory sensation. This is the moment when you have to stop yourself and move your hand away from your penis. You will probably lose part or all of your firm erection. Then, stimulate yourself again and stop. On the third time bring yourself to ejaculation. By this time you will have been able to stop twice and will have learned what you have to do in order not to ejaculate. You should take pride in having learned to control your ejaculation.

If you bring on an initial spurt or dribble, though not a full ejaculation, you have still gone too far. So, go back and practice, practice, practice until there is no doubt in your mind that you are able to prevent ejaculation by stopping the stimulation. If you do this with the proper mental attitude—that you have a learning difficulty and not a deep psychological or physical problem—you will successfully learn within a few weeks how to delay your ejaculation. You will no longer resort to antierotic diversion tactics, such as reciting the alphabet backwards from the letter "Z."

We say that it is a learning problem because we found that many men who have this problem learned, when they were younger, to masturbate and ejaculate very rapidly. That is, when they were in their early teens they would get aroused by looking at erotic pictures, having erotic thoughts or physical stimulation from clothing or the way they sat. Because they often didn't have the privacy or time for prolonged masturbation, they would go to the bathroom or under their covers and masturbate as quickly as possible before someone discovered them. Men have reported to us that these adolescent situations were carried over to the military where they had to relieve themselves in the shower or in their bunks as quickly as possible. This was because of the rarity of sexual partners in the military and the lack of privacy for slow autoerotic gratification.

This tendency to ejaculate as soon as possible may be reinforced, according to Kinsey, the great sex researcher, by what appears to be an instinctive desire in most male animals, to enter the female and ejaculate as soon as possible because they are at risk from predators during mating. If this is so, then it makes sense that human males have to *learn* to delay ejaculation because it may go against instinctual desires. You learn to do this by building confidence that you can stop when you want and ejaculate when you choose to. When you repeatedly try but cannot have any impact on controlling the ejaculation, especially if you ejaculate without any repetitive, rhythmic stimulation, then it is time to see a psychotherapist for further evaluation.

Erectile Difficulties

First of all, see your urologist. If the urologist deduces that there is nothing wrong with the physiological mechanisms, then the culprit is probably anxiety. You may have to see a sex therapist or a psychotherapist. But first, try our program here in the book because sometimes the anxiety may have a relatively simple cause. The erection failure may be based on a previous experience, that is, being with someone when you could not have the erection you wanted. At the time you may have been very tired, affected by too many drinks or medication, or burdened with a serious problem on your mind. These kinds of "situational" difficulties, usually due to anxiety, are fairly easy to overcome. You just have to realize that the sexual apparatus is very delicate and if you have the slightest anticipatory anxiety that you won't get an erection—you probably won't. You must reduce your anxiety by means of the exercises we have recommended in this book—fantasies, erotic thinking, stress reduction, and all the rest.

If your erectile difficulty is chronic, not just with one particular partner or on specific identifiable occasions, then you will have to do a good deal more digging to find the source of the problem. In all cases, begin with some self-analysis. Go for a walk in the park and try to figure out what happened when. When did you first start to have such difficulties? Can you achieve an erection if you masturbate? Do you have morning erections? Do you have erections with some partners but not with others? When you take this walk in the park to think about the personal circumstances of your erectile difficulties, it is important to sort out things with clarity. There are three main possibilities as to where the core of the problem lies:

- The problem began with and is limited to the present partner.
- The erectile problem seems to be extended to partners in general, but you can masturbate yourself to orgasm.
- The problem doesn't seem to be linked to partners because you can't get an erection even when you masturbate.

If you realize that your erectile difficulty is linked to your spouse or present lover, then you know that your relationship's problems have been brought to the bedroom. Perhaps you are subconsciously angry with your partner and want to withold your desire, your love, and your penis. In either case, sex therapy is probably not going to help at this time. You must first pick yourselves up and call a marriage or relationship counselor. Where the problem is in the penis, see the sex therapist or urologist—where the problem is in the heart or head, see the psychotherapist.

Now, if you can masturbate yourself to orgasm but you cannot obtain or maintain an erection with a partner, then the problem is not organic or physiological in nature. Because some interpersonal or other more deeply rooted factor is the cause, you should seek out the help of a psychotherapist or a sex therapist who is also qualified to work with emotional problems. As we have said before: Sex therapy has its limitations and the sex therapist must know the boundaries in order to be most effective. If you go to a sex therapist, and you have a problem that doesn't lend itself to an easy solution by simple exercises or learning or sexual literacy, then make sure the sex therapist is qualified to handle your emotional or physical problems. Usually, your local physician will be able to explain what training and qualifications in a person are needed to treat your problem.

Sometimes, if you have a sexual dysfunction *and* a marital problem, you can work on both at the same time with the marital counselor and the sex therapist cooperating. There are also sex therapists who are trained to do marital counseling, allowing you to see just one person. Make sure that they are well trained and highly recommended; begin by asking your physician for a referral.

The third type of erectile difficulty that men may experience may be the most intimidating of all. Here the man cannot obtain an erection at all, and the urologist says that there is nothing physically wrong. You may have taken and repeatedly failed the "postage stamp test" we discussed in Chapter 3 (placing attached postage stamps around the penis at night to see if an erection during sleep will break the stamps). Even in your dreams, then, the libido or sexual interest seem to be missing. If you know it's not caused by drugs, disease, or anything physical that the urologist can discover, what is left for you to do? Well, there are several things. First of all, we would suggest that you go back over this book carefully and work hard at *building interest*. Remember, you can build up your interest in sex—it's not all hormones and chemicals in the body. Sexual interest is mainly in your head, so use your head and focus more on sex through fantasy, reading erotic literature, watching erotic movies, and so forth. Direct your sex life in the direction you want to go by focussing in on the sexual roles and situations that always gave you the most stimulation and satisfaction.

There is also something you can do on the physical level. Several times a day—but, please, not in public—stroke your penis and testicles while engaging in your favorite erotic fantasies and memories. At other times, stroke your penis for the physical sensation without fantasizing, so you can focus all your attention on increasing sensations. Be imaginative. At the right times and places anoint your penis with various oils, gels, and creams. Have your fantasized lover or lovers give your penis a name, showering him with love and caresses as you soak in the bathtub, hot tub or spa. Be kind to him and love him as you should love yourself. Don't be bashful, let yourself go and enjoy some pleasure. You deserve it. But remember, this is not something that can change in one or two days. Be patient and keep at anything that brings you some results. Slowly, build up the small advances to the point where a decent erection is fairly sure.

Other men who do have erections are concerned that they are not as firm, as rigid as they once were. This may be due to poorer response to physical stimulation, to aging, or to weaker erotic context. What can you do? Look upon the situation as many professionals do with their professional training. They need continuing professional education to ensure that they keep up with current knowledge and skills. No less true for your penis. You must keep up its education as you get older because what may have aroused it to fantastic levels when you were younger may no longer be appropriate at this stage in your life. That is why fantasy is such a useful aid to sexual satisfaction. You can safely, in the privacy of your own imagination, experiment with ideas and situations and make-believe partners that may restore the old vitality to that semi-erect penis. You have to teach your penis to become excited again through your fantasies and other techniques learned from this book. You also need to, once again, become aware of those sensations associated with a growing erection while you practice building sexual desire. Do this on a regular basis, and be as faithful to it as you would be to a physical workout or diet regimen. Of course, improving your overall health condition may also help your sexual vitality.

Another problem we sometimes treat is dissatisfaction with the ability to maintain an erection. If a man loses his erection during coitus or oral sex it may be because some strong negative thought intruded. In other cases, it may be due to the man getting older and worrying about the physical strain of performing sex in the missionary position (the man on top of the woman). The physical effort of sex, for him, may overpower the pleasure that he is receiving. This is particularly true for men who allow themselves to get out of shape as they get older. In some cases, the loss of erection may be due to fears of physical exertion when they have a heart condition or severe asthma. In these cases, definitely see your physician.

But when the loss of erection appears to be the result of negative thinking or anxiety, then go back and practice the stress-reduction *and* the erotic-image-building exercises in our earlier chapters. If you are simply getting out of shape, *do something about it and don't complain.* While you embark on your exercise regimen, with consultation from your physician, try new positions with your partner that are less physically taxing for you. Let her get on top. She will enjoy it and so will you. While you are in this position, practice and increase the intensity of your most successful fantasies to help you out a bit. Being in the passive position, with someone making love to your body, could also help you to eradicate any possible negative thoughts or doubts about yourself. (If you have a female partner at this point who has practiced the love muscle exercises mentioned above, she can use this muscle to stimulate your penis if it begins to get soft while she is on top. Fantastic!) Also, don't forget that most men, as they get older, need more physical stimulation to both obtain and maintain an erection. The kind of psychogenic erection they were able to obtain as a teenager, when just holding the hand of a girl, is not likely to occur as he gets older. It is important that you communicate this to your partner as you get older, so that she doesn't interpret it as your loss of interest in her or that she is becoming unattractive.

Retarded Ejaculation

There are some men who report that they have no problem with erections and they are able to ejaculate either with a partner or through masturbation, but that it takes much longer than they want it to. That is, it may take so long that they get tired or even begin to lose interest in their sexual activity. They cannot ejaculate in a reasonable period of time and they begin to feel that they have to "work" at it. Sex then becomes a frustrating experience.

In many respects, this is analogous to the retarded orgasm in women that we talked about earlier in this chapter. The suggestions we made to women about varying the sexual conditions and fantasies until the right combination is found also applies to men. Increasing your erotic sex play will often help. Try, for example, oral sex, massage, masturbating in front of your partner while she also masturbates, vibrators, and so forth. Some couples swear by their VCRs. And especially for you men, we recommend varying the sexual positions during coitus until maximum stimulation to the penis is found. Position changes are less important for the woman because coitus usually provides more stimulation to a penis than to the clitoris. Also, there is a noticeable decrease in sensitivity for men who are sleepy or tired. So make sure you are full of energy and well rested before sex; you'll notice the difference. And make sure you don't drink or eat too much before sex! If the problem persists you should consult with a psychotherapist to learn why you are, subconsciously, so reluctant to ejaculate.

Lack of Desire

This is easy. Everything we said about the solutions to this problem for women at the beginning of this chapter also applies to men, although sometimes in slightly altered form. Read it again. Try what we say and learn to increase your level of desire through practice, practice, and more practice!

CHAPTER 9

What You and Your Partner Can Do for Each Other

Now that you have developed your erotic skills and you have tried to work through your problems by yourself, you may be dissatisfied with solo activity. You may feel that you could do much more if you try to work things out with a partner. Or, you may be one of the more fortunate people who have no sexual problems or deficiencies but want to help a beloved partner. In any case this chapter is for those people who have the kind of sexual problems that can be best worked on with company. For women, the main problems that we will cover in this chapter will be orgasmic difficulties and painful intercourse. For men, we will suggest ways that your partner can help you overcome the problems of premature ejaculation and erectile difficulties.

We must again emphasize that one cannot directly plunge into these "end of process" exercises with the hope of instant success without going through the many different stages and suggestions we made in previous chapters. Changing the patterns of sexual response to a more desired kind is not a quickie process. Time, patience, and a loving partner are most effective complements to the erotic mind-sets and relaxation skills mentioned in earlier chapters.

Orgasmic Response Difficulties

While it may come as a surprise to some readers, we have very little to say here about men helping women achieve orgasm. This is because the old notion that it is the man's responsibility to bring a woman to orgasm—and that if she doesn't have orgasms, it is the man's fault—is just plain rubbish. Women are much too knowledgeable and sophisticated today to be still willing to accept the old Victorian definitions of their sexuality. Women can increase their orgasmic responsiveness by themselves, after working through the relaxation and erotic exercises in the earlier chapters. That they may want to also try them with a partner is fine, provided that the partner himself (or herself) is no source of strain or stress to women with orgasmic difficulties.

Perhaps the most important thing a man can do to help a woman when she is having orgasmic difficulties is to make sure that he does not pressure the woman by asking her: "Are you coming?" or "How much longer do you think it will take?" or anything else that she may perceive not as concern, but as pressure. If he puts this pressure on her while she is showing him how she wants to be stimulated, this may not be too well received and is certainly not helpful.

There are some women who prefer the idea to develop their orgasmic responsiveness in the company of the ones they love. They may feel more sexually sensitive when with their lovers and more inhibited, due to conditioning, when alone. If this is what they choose to do, fine! The methods of self-pleasuring and self-stimulation mentioned in the last chapter can be used by such a couple.

We sincerely hope that the relaxation skills, erotic stimulations, and the use of vibrators, etc. has helped many have orgasms by themselves. But for some women, particularly those who want to have this experience with a lover only, some more work needs to be done. Even those women who are able to have orgasms by themselves may not be able to reach orgasm while their partners stimulate them or while having intercourse. (Please, please, don't get the idea that orgasms during intercourse are "better" or "more normal" than from other kinds of stimulation. They are all the same; only the aesthetics may be different.)

Stage One Exercises: Touching

What should the couple do? They should first make sure that the setting is private, attractive, comfortable, and warm. (It is very difficult to get turned on when you are chilled—even more so for men.) Make yourselves as relaxed as possible in as romantic a setting as you can arrange. Begin with lots of kissing and simple touching. The man must remember that the objective of these sessions is *not* to bring the woman to orgasm, but to create a set of conditions that will be repeated and intensified in future sessions. He should not look upon what goes on between them as "foreplay" because then he will expect it to lead to orgasm response during these sessions, which will confuse what should be happening. In these first few sessions, therefore, they should not go beyond simple kissing, hugging, and gentle touching in all those places of erotic sensitivity they discovered during the "body mapping" exercises in this book. This touching should not directly involve the clitoris, penis, or nipples.

These sensuous but non-sexual exercises are called *Sensate Focussing* discussed by the renowned sex therapist and educator, Dr. Helen Singer Kaplan. She suggests that in these exercises the couple should caress each other all over the body without touching each other's genitalia. After a few sessions of doing this, the woman and the man tend to build up the psychological confidence that intense sensual activity does not mean that the man will be groping for her clitoris right away and looking for that orgasmic response or that his penis must be ready to get up and perform. It is not only just the caressing of the body that is important during these sessions but also the practice of setting the right romantic mood for their future sessions. After the first couple of sessions the couple should bring into play all of this book's tools for sexual stimulation, including fantasy, erotic imagery, beautiful scents, and so forth. But the couple must rely on self-control to ensure that they *don't* touch the genitals, or even the nipples, for several more sessions. How many sessions? That you must learn for yourself. For a start, try to have these sensate focus sessions at least a few times a week for two or three weeks. Then, the two of you should talk it over to see if either of you have any doubts about moving on to the next stage. When you are both convinced, then do it—but again, keep that self-control and wait until the next day.

It is the term *self-control* that is so important in developing these skills. One has to learn the skills and confidence to take control over one's own sex life before one can be happier in his or her sexual relationship. Do not confuse self-control with the inability to let go of emotions and feelings when they are called for. We believe that self-control is an active force in our lives as opposed to the passive reactive behavior that so many women (and men) believe is the right way to behave. In a sense, you can look at what we mean by self-control as the precursor and then partner of self-assertiveness. And, this self-control is also an aid in building trust in your partner—a prerequisite for letting go during the orgasmic response.

Stage Two Exercises: Exploration

We call the next stage of sessions *exploratory.* That is because we want you to go no further than exploring each other's genitals by looking, touching, tasting, and even smelling. The man can explore the folds of his partner's vagina, the beauty of her clitoris, and the surrounding areas just as well as the woman will explore the beauty of her partner's penis and testicles and other parts of his body. You will not be trying to stimulate your partner during these sessions, but, again, making each other feel very comfortable and non-pressured when genitals are explored and made to feel a most natural and comfortable part of the body. It is very important during these second-stage sessions that you first review the first stage of just touching, hugging, and kissing each other without touching the genitals.

In this second level of sessions, you will return to your romantic, secure setting to recreate those successful and pleasurable non-genital touching sessions for a comfortable period of time (but more than just a few minutes), before moving on to the exploration of each other's genitals. This exploration is not clinical exploration, and all "body mapping" of the most erotic parts should already have been learned by yourself. This exploration is a learning experience, in interaction with others, to see what is most stimulating in these kinds of situations. You will discover that what is or isn't stimulating when by yourself, may not be the case when you are with a partner. During these exploring sessions, each has to play an adult version of "show and tell." That is, they have to tell each other where they would like to be explored and show the other person where the finger, hand, or tongue should be placed. Don't assume that your partner is a mind reader. We can assure you that this will not be the case and that missed communications based on such assumptions can be very destructive in a relationship. For example, a man may want his anus to be touched while his partner may wrongly assume that he will find it distasteful. You would be amazed at how often we find, even after many years of a sexual relationship, that a couple really doesn't know each other's likes and dislikes. Sometimes people don't even know their own because they have never explored their own bodies in detail or allowed a lover to do so with the systematic, leisurely approach we recommend.

It may happen that in the course of exploring each other's bodies, one or even both of you may have orgasms. That is O.K. as long as it was not the intent of one partner to stimulate the other to an orgasm. It is very important to build the confidence in each partner that the orgasm should occur when they are ready for it, that is, when they are in control of their own sexual outcomes.

Stage Three Exercises: Stimulation

When both partners feel that they want to go on to achieve orgasm in a couple situation, they may begin the final set of exercises. Again, they must build upon the successful sensations and confidence-building of the first two stages. For a number of sessions—*whether or not one or both of them reaches orgasm during a session*—they should begin each session with kissing, hugging, and non-genital touching, followed by a period of pleasurable exploring. Only *then* should they introduce the new element of deliberate sexual stimulation. Now, depending on whether it is the woman or the man who has the problem in reaching orgasm, the couple must temporarily focus more on the problem partner.

Assuming that the problem partner is the woman (since statistically she is more likely to have a problem), the man should concentrate on using his fingers and/or tongue in those moves and pressures that he has learned to be most effective in stimulating his partner. As a rule, we would suggest that he does not try to bring her to climax with his penis at this stage. For most women, this is the least effective way for clitoral stimulation and so failure to reach orgasm might reinforce her old doubts about being at all able to have an orgasm.

Instead, first build up a pattern of success with easier methods such as manual or oral stimulation—or even with a vibrator. Make sure that the man uses the vibrator on the woman, if she uses one, so that it is a couple act and not a solo one. Then, in a loving and expectant manner help the woman build excitement until she reaches her orgasm. If at any time, however, the woman feels that she is losing interest or that the pleasurable sensation has turned to an uncomfortable one, she should communicate this to her partner and they should stop striving for her orgasm during that session. It would not be psychologically wise for her to work against what her body feels and then to fail.

Both members of the couple must be very patient during this process because sometimes it takes a very long time before a non-orgasmic woman is able to reach orgasm in this manner. The couple must not get so discouraged or anxious that they forget to recreate the successful steps of past sessions during this period. They must use the initial touching and exploring as a means of building up the erotic repertoire as well as continuing the education of the body-mind in sexual responsiveness. So, if it doesn't work the first time, try the next time and keep building these sensitivities and skills. If after a few weeks there is still no orgasm but the woman notices progress in the form of increasing desire or sensitivity, be patient and continue on. If, on the other hand, she feels that there is no progress or that she may even be retrogressing, then it is time for her to get evaluated by a sex therapist to find out if there is anything else wrong that she is not aware of.

No Orgasm During Intercourse

There are some women who may not have had any difficulty achieving orgasm by themselves or with their partner's help, manually or orally. There might even be those who were not previously orgasmic, but now are, after following our programs and advice. In either case these women may now want to have an orgasm during coitus. It is still necessary, for either kind of woman, to go through the former stages we have just outlined to insure that orgasm without penetration is achieved fairly easily. At that point, the couple may begin a new set of sessions that will introduce this new element of attempting to reach orgasm during intercourse.

Let us here emphasize the fact that some women will never be able to have an orgasm by the action of their partner's penis moving in and out. So what? This does not mean that there is anything wrong with either person, with their love for each other, or with their sexual skill. It is simply that the anatomy of one or another or both does not lend itself to the specific kind of stimulation needed by the woman to have that orgasm without some additional aid from fingers, a vibrator, or whatever. We will show you how to achieve orgasm during coitus, but do not get any false ideas that an orgasm during penetration or simultaneous orgasms during intercourse is going to set fireworks off and bells ringing. The most important thing is for each of you to be able to please and pleasure your partner in the most loving way that is desired.

How does one learn to transfer the ability to reach orgasm outside of intercourse to achieving orgasm during intercourse? First of all, it is crucial that you precede any coitus with previous stages of *touching, exploration, and stimulation.* This is to recall in your mind the previous successes you have had and all the control you have learned over your sexual responsiveness. This time, however, the woman's partner should not stimulate her to orgasm but to a point very close to it. It is necessary for the woman to signal the man when she has reached this point, a sensation she will have learned in all the previous situations when she had an orgasm by herself or with a partner. At this special moment the man should insert his penis inside his wife or lover—making sure there is sufficient lubrication to prevent any discomfort or pain during penetration.

Which position should they use? Many women find that orgasm during intercourse is best facilitated when the man enters them from the rear—not in the anus but the vagina. This is most comfortably done when the woman is crouching on her hands and knees on the bed and the man is on his knees in back of her. For some men, it is easier if they are standing on the floor while the woman is crouching on the bed. After he enters her, she can either reach under, or he can reach around to stimulate the clitoris, which is more easily exposed in this position. The motions and rhythm of the clitoral stimulation can easily be synchronized to the movement of the penis. This will increase the psychological stimulation for some women, who may then associate the thrusts with the more pleasurable clitoral stimulation. The man or woman might also stimulate the clitoris while there is little or no thrusting of the penis until the woman feels that she is about to come. At this point the man should resume his thrusting while his finger, or hers, is stimulating her to orgasm.

After a few lovemaking sessions where manual stimulation brings her to orgasm while the penis is thrusting in and out, the couple can try a variation in which she ceases the manual stimulation an instant before coming to allow penile stimulation alone to trigger the orgasm. For some women, this will work; others will find that they still need the aid of a finger. Again, this is only due to anatomical structural differences and should be of no consequence.

If you are one of those women who can achieve orgasm through the movement of the penis a second or two after stopping manual stimulation, then you can probably eliminate the time lag in succeeding lovemaking sessions until one day you may find that you don't need manual stimulation at all during intercourse. If, however, you are one of the majority of women who need a little help, relax and enjoy it. Incorporate such stimulation in imaginative and innovative ways in your lovemaking in the secure knowledge that you can have the orgasm when you want to!

Many couples want variation in positions, and there certainly is no limit except for your imagination. That is, any position in which the man or the woman is able to use a hand and easily stimulate the clitoris during intercourse may be used as long as it is pleasurable to both partners and the same *transferring* of manual to penile triggering of the orgasm may be attempted by the couple. Helen Singer Kaplan has called this transferral process *the bridge*. It not only bridges the gap between auto-erotic stimulation and orgasm during coitus, but it also helps strengthen the bond between the two people in a loving relationship.

Paradoxically, the most common position, the so-called missionary position with the man on top of the woman, is often the least conducive to helping the woman have an orgasm during intercourse. This is not only due to the fact that her clitoris may get little stimulation from his penis in this position but also because it is more difficult to stimulate the clitoris with his or her finger. Therefore, because of mostly anatomical differences, many women will not be able to have orgasms brought about solely by the male using only his thrusting penis. This should not be of any concern to women. Orgasms brought on by a thrusting penis, while the man is on top, are not more satisfying orgasms, not more pleasurable, and not more natural. If a women wants to believe that they are, she may perceive that they are better, but orgasms in the missionary position should be considered one possible way, but not the only way to satisfying sex.

For most women, another position may help them achieve orgasm while the penis is inside of them. In this position they sit on top of the male (facing him) with their knees on the bed or floor for easier control of movement. They can readily stimulate the clitoris while moving up and down with the penis inside or they can easily stimulate the clitoris by rubbing the pelvis forward and back—toward his face and then back toward his toes. This movement while the penis is inside will provide much stimulation to both partners. Of course, the woman is fully in control in this position, and the man is usually lying back very passively. This may either bother or excite some men but is very useful when the man is tired and the woman is raring to go!

Whatever positions the couple try, it is very helpful if the woman recalls those fantasies that have been successful for her in the past, when she was using them to bring herself to orgasm. There is nothing wrong with a woman (or a man) who uses fantasy during intercourse to help heighten sexual excitement.

One technique that might be very helpful in enabling women to have orgasms during intercourse without the aid of manual stimulation is for them to go through a "learning" stage. During a lovemaking session, they do not engage in any motion while the penis is inside. Instead, a woman should bring herself to orgasm with a small vibrator (such as the Eroscillator we described in Chapter 5) with the penis remaining inside. Because the vibrator is so much more intense than manual stimulation for some women, they much more easily associate the orgasm with the feeling of the penis inside and can learn in just a few sessions to abandon the use of the vibrator and have just the penile thrusting bring them to orgasm. Try it—it might work for you. If not, you will still have fun trying! And never forget that sex *should* be fun and not something you have to work at. So, all through these exercises, try to introduce lightness and fun along with love and patience.

Going Beyond Orgasm

What do we mean by "beyond orgasm"? For one thing, there are some women who may be having orgasms, that is, they recognize some different and pleasurable sensations followed by a relaxation period, but they wonder if they are having the real thing. This sense of "missed orgasm" is probably due to an unrealistic expectation that some women develop because of the dramatic presentation of orgasmic responses in the mass media. The earth and the sky seem to move for women in television and movies suggesting some fabulous and overpowering sort of orgasmic response. A woman who believes what she sees or reads in the mass media might be having orgasms but they just don't register to her as the kind of pleasurable responses she *thinks* she should have. For those women who have orgasms but feel they are not "strong" or "intense" enough, we say that it is your perception of your response that can make you enjoy it more.

You must change yourself rather than somehow changing the physiological nature of the orgasm itself. How do you do this? By repeating and expanding the kinds of sexual sensitivity exercises and skills we have mentioned in the earlier chapters of this book. If you are now able to have orgasms this does not mean that you have completed your sexual skills training. You have reached a wonderful level of sexual satisfaction but you now should incorporate your new knowledge and skills into heightening the awareness and pleasurability of your orgasmic response. Remember: Practice! Practice! Practice! Enjoy your sexual activities to the fullest, but not always and only to reach orgasm. Repeat and expand upon many of the suggestions in this book to make the entire lovemaking session as pleasurable as possible for both of you. You can become a virtuoso of your own sexual responses, if you so desire.

Painful Intercourse

Once again, if you women have any pain at all during intercourse, see a gynecologist. While men rarely experience pain related to sexual intercourse, they should see their urologists or physicians as soon as they experience any mysterious pain or discomfort.

If your gynecologist says that nothing is physically wrong, then you and your partner can try what we recommend here along with whatever other exercises or recommendations are made to you by your doctor. If it appears to you—and your physician agrees—that the reasons for the pain are probably psychogenic in origin, that is, you are still not able to relax enough, then try some more work of the kind we have suggested in this book.

There are situations where there may be nothing physically wrong; you are fully able to relax, greatly desirous of your partner entering you, gushing with lubrication, have no psychological problems inhibiting you, yet one or both of you experience pain or discomfort. One cause could be the anatomical mismatch of a male partner who is "too well endowed" to fit easily into a woman's vagina. In other words, the man's penis may be a little too long or too thick for comfort. What are you going to do, if you believe that this is your situation?

In all probability, nothing more radical will be necessary than to try different positions with your partner until one is found that is comfortable for the two of you. Sometimes, the solution is a simple change like the woman sitting on top of the man as if she were riding a horse (English Saddle, not Western Saddle). In this position, many women are able to control the extent of penetration by moving down on the penis only as far as they feel comfortable. For other couples, the male may try a position where he enters his female partner from the rear (not into the anus, but into the vagina), so that the buttocks of the female act as a cushion to prevent deep penetration.

What are some of the other ways? For one, when the woman prefers the man to be on top it is possible for her to control the depth of penetration to some extent by the flexing of her legs as she places them around her partner. As many of you know from personal experience, the closer a woman brings her knees toward her chest or face during intercourse, the easier it becomes for the man to thrust deeply inside of her. Therefore, a woman who experiences pain or discomfort because of the size of her partner's penis may want to experiment with just the right angle that would eliminate the pressure or pain. For some couples, the use of a pillow under the behind of the woman may be more comfortable; for other couples, a pillow under the man with the woman on top, may give her maximum control over the depth of penetration.

If these suggestions still don't work, you might try a thick doughnut or bagel made from a sponge-like material that is placed around the penis and used as a cushion. Remember that all of these suggestions are only for pain or discomfort due to anatomical differences. Make sure a gynecologist says that everything else is O.K.

Vaginismus

For some women, the pain that they experience may be due to something a little more complicated and resistant to change: vaginismus. As we said in Chapter 8, some women experience pain upon penetration because the vaginal muscles have tightened up so much that the opening becomes too narrow for the penis to enter comfortably. Vaginismus involves an involuntary constriction of the vaginal muscles and some of these women cannot even use tampons. Dr. Helen Singer Kaplan, has elaborated upon a method whereby the partner can help a woman who has this problem. First, there should be a relatively long period of time set aside for the man to pleasure the woman. That is, he should spend a lot of time kissing her, hugging, touching all over her body, teasing her, and making her as sexually aroused as he knows how. When it seems that she is really getting turned on, he should then try to insert his pinky finger into her vagina, using K-Y or a good lubricant if needed. It may not work the first evening he tries, and it may take a few days or even a couple of months, but, eventually, he will be able to penetrate with his pinky without her feeling pain or pressure.

The man should continue this process on subsequent nights until he is able to get a thumb in and, later, two fingers. (Make sure you men keep your nails clean and trimmed!) By that time, she very likely will be relaxed enough for him to attempt penis penetration. But if it doesn't work out that night and he cannot get his penis inside, don't either of you make an issue out of it. Repeat the process of the lengthy pleasuring sessions—increasing the penetration from pinky to two fingers and always making sure that there is sufficient lubrication. Eventually, with enough patience, love, and sensitivity to the woman's responses—plus her continuing the relaxation exercises mentioned earlier in this book—the couple will be successful at overcoming vaginismus and achieving coitus.

Some sex therapists recommend the use of dilators (see Chapter 8) to aid in the relaxing of the vaginal muscles. We usually don't. We believe that when a woman has a partner, there is much to be gained by overcoming this problem within a mutually satisfying relationship and without the aid of artificial devices. If a woman does not have a partner to help her, she then can use the dilators as we described in Chapter 8. While we still feel that the human touch is the best, if your gynecologist recommends dilators, and if you and your partner prefer them to the fingers method, by all means use them! Some couples may even find their use sexually arousing.

Sometimes, all this loving effort by the man to help his partner overcome her problem, ironically creates new problems. A couple in treatment came into the office and the husband said: "Dr. Ruth, we did everything exactly as you told us, and your advice was absolutely wonderful. But now, I have a problem too. Since the last time we saw you, I was able to get two of my fingers inside my wife's vagina fairly easily. Although she felt a slight pressure, she said it felt fine. We were both very excited. I got on top and just as I was about to place my penis inside of her—I lost my erection! This has never happened to me before when I was sexually excited. Then, last night, we were trying again, and went through the whole process. Just as I was about to enter her vagina, I ejaculated on the outside before I could get my penis inside. This too never happened before, unless my wife was stimulating my penis. What is happening to me?"

Although he was obviously upset and concerned, the advice given to him was simple and short: "Don't worry about it!" This does happen to some men—this very temporary loss of erection or premature ejaculation. They have concentrated so much for so long on getting their partners aroused, that they lose track of their own degree of sexual arousal (or lack of it) at the critical moment. We notice this to be particularly true of men who intellectualize too much during the lovemaking process instead of just going with their feelings. Of course, this doesn't happen to all men in the course of trying to help their partners, but if you happen to be one of them, don't become overly concerned. Just go to sleep and try again the next morning or whenever. Of course, since the woman was highly aroused at the time this happened, he could still bring her to orgasm manually, orally, or in whatever manner pleases her—including the use of a vibrator. So, first bring her to orgasm before you go to sleep and try again the next day. Your problem is clearly related to your intellectually concentrating on helping your partner, and it is very unlikely that such occurrences signal an oncoming chronic problem.

We cannot stress the importance of patience enough, both on the part of the man and the woman, because solving the problems of vaginismus sometimes takes longer than we would hope. But keep at it. Once there is penetration by the fingers and then the penis, there should no longer be any pain or uncomfortable pressure for the woman. If there still is, by all means go back to your gynecologist.

We once had this interesting couple as patients who were happily married for years. When they had "sex" he rubbed his penis against her abdomen and ejaculated. He then gave her an orgasm manually. Without penetration, they had never consummated their marriage. The woman now wanted to become pregnant, but they knew that he would have to place his penis inside of her in order for the fertilization to take place. Even though the woman could have orgasms, vaginismus would not permit his penis to enter her. Regular orgasms do not mean that vaginal muscles will relax enough for penetration. In their case, after a period of sex therapy, nature was able to take its course. His penis found its way in and nine months later she gave birth to a healthy son!

Premature Ejaculation

In the last chapter, we discussed the different ways and the different techniques that a man should use to learn how to *control* his ejaculation, so that it happens when *he* wants it to and not otherwise. We don't like the phrase "to delay ejaculation" (even though most therapists still use that phrase) because too often men and their female partners get the notion that there is a "natural" time for ejaculation to take place. The man then feels he should use artificial devices like thinking about income taxes, in order to fool Mother Nature. This could be a destructive way of looking at the situation.

We prefer to see the problem of premature ejaculation as a *learning* difficulty—one must unlearn one set of responses and learn a new set. Only rarely do we find a situation in which premature ejaculation is some kind of a deep-rooted emotional or psychiatric problem. Of course, many men are very troubled by this problem and it can have its emotional impact on a man or a couple. Nonetheless, the resolution of the problem is, by and large, still a matter of learning. Here in this chapter, the issue is how can a partner help a man learn these new responses and overcome premature ejaculation.

If a man with this problem is not living with someone in a loving relationship, it is very important that he do what we suggested in the last chapter, working by himself for a few weeks before he tries out his new skills with a partner. It is especially important that he should avoid intercourse during this period if he is not in a stable love relationship. The reason for this is that just in case there are any elements in nonpermanent relationships that may be affecting his premature ejaculation difficulties, they should not be allowed to interfere with the learning process. He needs the maximum opportunity to recognize, by himself—without the distraction of a casual sex partner—those premonitory sensations that he experiences just before that "point of no return" and ejaculation.

During these few weeks, even though he can give any female partner he is with as many manual or oral orgasms as she wants, it would be advisable if he were to concentrate only on his learning experience. Although he first has to learn this control by himself, we realize that it is important for his partner not to be frustrated, rejected, or left out. The couple should therefore agree that after his self-stimulation exercises, even those to the point of ejaculation, he will still pleasure her and stimulate her to her orgasm without intercourse. It is important that this is done *after—not before or during his important self-stimulation exercises.* After a few weeks of self-therapy, then he will be able to have his partner work with him. The self-stimulation exercises can move on to the couple-oriented exercises when the man is successfully able to hold off his ejaculation for a reasonable period of time. If he has not been able to learn this by himself, there is very little point in trying to do this with a casual partner. It usually won't work. Almost all men, however, can learn to control the time of ejaculation by the stop-and-start technique we outlined in the last chapter.

Now, if a couple comes to therapy together, or if a man is in a stable, loving relationship, the situation is a little different. There, we can skip the solely auto-erotic exercises and have his wife or significant other work with him from the start. Even a man who feels very comfortable with his partner may want to try to learn the self-control process by himself. Again, there should be no intercourse during these learning sessions.

Let's begin! The couple should be in a comfortable and secure setting where they are not likely to be interrupted or distracted by children, telephone, the dog wanting to go outside, or anything like that. Once they are ready, the woman should begin by providing him with a mild form of sexual stimulation. More powerful stimulation, such as oral sex, may prevent him from recognizing the premonitory sensations. That is, if the stimulation is too strong, the premonitory stage may pass by so quickly that he could not tell her to stop the stimulation in time. Any premature ejaculation during these sessions would only reinforce his belief that he is unable to control himself. The partner has to go slowly in these exercises, remembering that she is not trying to be as sexy or skillful a lover as possible, but someone in tune with the man's learning process. Her husband is developing a new pattern of responding to stimulation—one in which he is able to control himself.

The wife or partner must also concentrate on what she is doing because once he says "Stop," she must instantly stop her stimulation. If she has her mind on something else or she's fantasizing, she might not be able to stop at the right moment. The woman is not supposed to excite her partner as much as possible, only sufficiently for him to maintain his erection. She must be alert to doing exactly as he tells her to do. Usually this is not an erotic experience for a woman. It is, more importantly, a helping experience to allow the man to recognize his premonitory sensations as well as helping him by discussing those sensations. Her role is to help make him even more acutely aware of what they are through his verbalizing these sensations with his partner. He does not have to discuss these sensations every time he tells her to stop, but at the early stages of these exercises it will help him concentrate on self-knowledge and self-analysis.

When the man tells his partner to stop the stimulation, he may lose some of the firmness of his erection. This is natural for some men, particularly as they get a little older, and nothing to worry about. It merely means that his partner will need to give him a bit more stimulation before his penis regains firmness and he can again reach the point just before that moment of inevitability. Again, he should tell her to stop as soon as he realizes that he is at that point and she should do so immediately. To refresh your memory: The moment just before the ejaculation is inevitable is that point at which the orgasm is beginning but ejaculation has not yet occurred. When he learns to recognize it in time and have the stimulation cease immediately, the ejaculation will not occur.

Why is it that so many men seem unaware of this momentary lag between the beginning of the orgasmic sensation and its heightening during ejaculation? It is not too difficult to understand. For most men, orgasm is the goal of sexual activity, not the sensations along the way. These men have never been trained to become sensitive to the different sensations of the orgasm and are largely unaware that there is still time to control the process. These exercises are a learning process, and most men will not pick up this new skill of self-control in just one or two sessions. When the man does ejaculate unintentionally, talk to him about how it felt just before the onset of the orgasmic stage. Turn the minor failure into a major lesson so that he can better recognize these sensations the next time.

How many times should a man try these exercises before attempting to control his ejaculation during intercourse? This is difficult to say for all cases. Minimally, you should have at least three successful sessions of exercises. At the end of each successful session the man should attain full ejaculation when *he decides the time is right.* These ejaculations should still be outside of the vagina, with his partner stimulating him as before. And he shouldn't forget to give his wife special pleasuring and orgasms to reward her for her patience and effort.

After the man feels that he has gained stop-and-start control over his ejaculation, he is ready to try to maintain this control during coitus. The woman must first be fully ready, physically and psychologically, so that nothing interferes with the man's concentration. He won't be able to focus on applying the learning process if his wife or lover feels uncomfortable during coitus.

For these exercises, the woman should be on top, moving up and down while her husband or significant other lies there passively. With less physical effort, he has maximum opportunity to concentrate on preorgasmic sensations. As soon as he becomes aware of the premonitory sensations, he should immediately tell her to stop her movements until he no longer feels an urge to ejaculate. He should keep his penis inside of her during this pause and he will soon be ready for her to resume her stimulating movements. After practicing this stopping and starting a few times, he can choose *when* to ejaculate and should tell her to continue what she is doing until he does reach his full climax. In the meantime, she must concentrate on helping her husband or partner to learn this control, rather than trying to bring herself to orgasm through her movements. After he is finished with his orgasm, he should bring her to orgasm manually or orally. During these sessions, the man should not try to pleasure her before he reaches climax because this will distract him from recognizing the premonitory sensations.

One effective variation of this same position involves the woman, on top, using her *pubococcygeal* (PC) muscle, as described in the last chapter. For some women, tightening and relaxing this muscle to stimulate her partner's penis is much easier and less tiring than moving their bodies up and down with the penis inside.

Many women learn how to take a soft penis and place it inside their vaginas, using the PC muscle to stimulate it to erection. Some writers have called this "stuffing." This is a particularly useful skill for the woman to know as her husband gets a little older, because it becomes increasingly likely that a man's erection will subside more quickly and take longer to become firm again. If his penis goes soft inside of her, it might easily slip out when either of them resumes motion. If the woman has learned to use her PC muscle skillfully, she can stimulate the soft penis and bring it to full erection without either of them having to move. This skill saves the couple from having to repeat all the external stimulation needed before an erect penis can re-enter the vagina. Many men report that stimulation via the PC muscle is fantastic, so it's a valuable skill for the wives and lovers of men of all ages.

After a few sessions where his partner helped him start and stop a few times before coming to full orgasm, the man is now ready to try this self-control in the male superior or missionary position. During this stage of learning the man must again learn to recognize those sensations that immediately precede his orgasm. He must stop his own thrusting at the right moment. He cannot just tell her to stop because now he is doing the work. Of course, she must stop immediately if she were moving her hips in rhythm with his thrusting. Therefore, he must tell her to stop at the instant he recognizes that the orgasm is near or she must be supersensitive to his motions so that she will stop as soon as he does. In most cases, the man will be able to resume his thrusting again just after he feels those pleasant sensations subside.

The stopping and starting gets easier, more second-nature, with each time and after each session. Since learning to control the timing of his orgasm is a little more difficult while the man is on top and more active, it is difficult to predict the number of times he will have to do this until premature ejaculation is no longer a problem. So, practice, practice, practice! Because the solution is a skill, the problem of premature ejaculation usually does not return. If it does—practice and more practice.

Erectile Difficulties

What can a woman do to help her significant other if he has difficulties in either obtaining or maintaining an erection? First, make sure he has seen a urologist to rule out any physiological problems or to see if he has been affected by medications for hypertension or some other condition. Once we know that there is nothing physically wrong, then the male should carefully study what we have said in the last chapter about ruling out intrusive psychological factors or conditions. He should make sure that the problem is not the relationship, his current life situation or some other situational circumstances that may be causing the erectile difficulties.

Also, the couple should examine their lovemaking environment to make sure that it is as comfortable, secure, and romantic as reasonably possible. This environment must be non-stressful, and one that both are completely satisfied with.

Once the couple has ruled out both physical and situational sources of the difficulty, then the issue likely revolves around the erotic stimulation necessary to obtain and maintain an erection. To work with this issue, draw upon all the erotic knowledge and skills that you have picked up in the preceding chapters and apply them in the bedroom. Use your collective imagination to enhance your sexual union with fantasizing, hot tubs, bubble baths, visual erotic stimuli, vibrators, and whatever. Do it with enthusiasm and tremendous *joie de vivre!* Those erectile difficulties will not stand a chance.

An Old-fashioned Conclusion

At a time when so many people do not have ongoing stable sexual relationships, we increased our desire to learn how to be optimal sexual partners. We strongly advocate accomplishing this sexual competence within a stable relationship such as marriage. We are not only considering the dangers of disease and the psychological discomforts of loneliness, but also the old-fashioned and everlasting needs for love, emotional security, and family. The myth of the joyous swinging single who has the most fantastic sex is precisely that: a myth.

Only in stable relationships do people have the optimal opportunities and emotional security to truly develop sexual skills and pleasures. Only a solid couple can help each other achieve maximum erotic stimulation and satisfaction.

Never forget that the best sex results from a lifelong process of learning. People change and grow, and the relationships between love, affection, sensuality, and eroticism change at different ages and time periods. If you allow yourself the right to have maximum erotic pleasure and you are willing to work at this learning process, sex can become better and better as you get older. And the older you become, the better lover you will be. Continue to learn and continue to love!

Recommended Reading

Barbach, Lonnie G. *For Yourself: The Fulfillment of Female Sexuality.* New York: New American Library, 1976.

———. *Women Discover Orgasm: A Therapist's Guide to a New Treatment Approach.* New York: Macmillan, 1980.

Benson, Herbert. *The Relaxation Response.* New York: Morrow, 1975. London: Collins, 1976.

Brecher, Edward M. *The Sex Researchers.* Boston: Little, Brown, 1980. London: Andre Deutsch, 1970.

——. *Love, Sex, and Aging.* Boston & London: Little, Brown, 1984.

Brothers, Joyce. *The Successful Woman: How You Can Have a Career, a Husband, and a Family—and Not Feel Guilty About It.* New York & London: Simon and Schuster, 1988.

Calderone, Mary S., and Eric W. Johnson. *The Family Book About Sexuality.* New York: Harper and Row, 1981. London: Harper Collins, 1990.

Comfort, Alex. *The Joy of Sex.* New York: Crown, 1972. London: Quartet, 1976.

Dodson, Betty. *Sex for One: The Joy of Self-loving.* New York: Harmony, 1987.

Fowkes, Charles (ed.). *The Illustrated Kama Sutra: Ananga-Ranga-Perfumed Garden.* New York: Exeter Books, 1987.

Friday, Nancy. *My Secret Garden: Women's Sexual Fantasies.* New York: Trident, 1973. London: Quartet, 1979.

———. *Forbidden Flowers: More Women's Sexual Fantasies.* New York: Pocket Books, 1975.

———. *Men in Love.* New York: Delacorte, 1982. London: Hutchinson, 1980.

Kaplan, Helen S. *The New Sex Therapy: Active Treatment of Sexual Dysfunctions.* New York: Brunner/Mazel, 1974. London: Baillière, 1980.

———. *Disorders of Sexual Desire.* New York: Simon and Schuster, 1979. Cambridge University Press, 1987.

———. *The Evaluation of Sexual Disorders: Psychological and Medical Aspects.* New York: Brunner/Mazel, 1983.

———. *Sexual Aversion, Sexual Phobias, and Panic Disorder.* New York: Brunner/Mazel, 1987.

Kinsey, A. C., W. B. Pomeroy, and C. E. Martin. *Sexual Behavior in the Human Male.* Philadelphia: W. B. Saunders, 1948.

——— and P. H. Gebhard. *Sexual Behavior in the Human Female.* Philadelphia: W. B. Saunders, 1953.

Masters, William H., and Virginia E. Johnson. *Human Sexual Inadequacy.* Boston & London: Little, Brown, 1970.

Montague, Ashley. *Touching: The Human Significance of the Skin.* New York: Columbia University Press, 1986. London: Harper and Row, 1986.

Siegel, Bernard S. *Love, Medicine and Miracles.* New York· Harper and Row, 1988. London: Century, 1986.

Silverstein, Charles. *Man to Man: Gay Couples in America.* New York: William Morrow, 1981.

——— and Edmund White. *The Joy of Gay Sex.* New York: Crown, 1977.

Sisley, Emily, and Bertha Harris. *The Joy of Lesbian Sex.* New York: Crown, 1977.

Smith, B. *Twentieth-Century Masters of Erotic Art.* New York: Crown, 1980.

Weil, Andrew. *The Natural Mind: A New Way of Looking at Drugs and the Higher Consciousness.* Boston: Houghton Mifflin, 1972. London: Cape, 1973.

Westheimer, Ruth. *Dr. Ruth's Guide to Good Sex.* New York: Warner, 1983. London: W.H. Allen, 1987.

———. *Dr. Ruth's Guide for Married Lovers.* New York: Warner, 1986.

——— and Louis Lieberman. *Sex and Morality: Who Is Teaching Our Sex Standards?* New York: Harcourt Brace Janovich, 1988.

Zilbergeld, Bernie. *Male Sexuality: A Guide to Sexual Fulfillment.* Boston: Little, Brown, 1978.